SECRETS to LOSE TOXIC BELLY FAT!

Heal Your Sick Metabolism Using State-Of-The-Art Medical Testing and Treatment With Detoxification, Diet, Lifestyle, Supplements, and Bioidentical Hormones

USE THE SECRET ACTION PLAN TO:

- **Overcome Sick Metabolism and Lose Stubborn Belly Fat!**
- **Learn about Prevention of Heart Disease, Cancer, and Diabetes!**
- **Balance Your Hormones!**
  - Sex Hormones: Estrogen, Progesterone, and Testosterone.
  - Adrenal Hormones: Cortisol and DHEA.
  - Thyroid, Insulin, Leptin, Ghrelin, and Growth Hormone.
- **Treat the Hormonal Deficiencies of Menopause and Andropause!**
- **Optimize Estrogen Metabolism to Prevent Breast/Prostate Cancer!**
- **Balance Your Neurotransmitters!**
  - Serotonin.
  - Acetylcholine.
  - Noradrenalin.
  - Dopamine.
  - GABA.
- **Begin to Reverse Chronic Degenerative Diseases!**
  - Metabolic Syndrome.
  - Impaired Immunity.
  - Impaired Digestion.
  - Bacterial, Viral, Parasite, and Yeast Infections.
  - Chronic Fatigue.
  - Nerve and Brain Disorders.
  - Auto-Immune Disorders (Arthritis, Allergies, Lupus, M.S).

I0414958

Look great!
Feel great!
Lose weight!
Have better sex!

Book Six in the Series, "Bioidentical Hormones."

J.M. Swartz M.D.
Y.L. Wright M.A.

First Edition

Copyright © 2012 by J.M. Swartz M.D. and Y.L. Wright M.A.

All Rights Reserved. No part of this document may be reproduced without written consent from the authors.

Published by Lulu.com in the United States

ISBN: 978-1-105-81198-2

Printed in the United States of America

MEDICAL DISCLAIMER:
     The following text is for general information only. It contains the opinions and ideas of the authors. Careful attention has been paid to insure the accuracy of the information, but the authors and the publisher cannot assume responsibility for the validity or consequences of its use. The intention of this book is to provide helpful information. This information is not intended to diagnose or treat any disease. This book is sold with the understanding that the authors and publisher are not rendering medical, health, or any other professional services. See your medical or health professional concerning any health concerns or before following any suggestions made in this book or drawing inferences from it. The authors and publisher specifically disclaim all responsibility for any liability, loss, or risk incurred as a direct or indirect consequence of using this book's contents. Any use of the information found in this book is the sole responsibility of the reader. Any dietary, nutrient, hormone, and medication suggestions found in this book are to be followed only under the supervision of a medical doctor or endocrine specialist. The authors receive no compensation from endorsement of any products or companies mentioned in this book.

DEDICATION:
     This book is written for you. If even one person finds their way out of chronic disease and suffering into health, it has been worth it.

Read all of the books in the "Bioidentical Hormones" series:
This book is the sixth book in the series, "Bioidentical Hormones." Our mission is to bring you the latest scientific information about hormone optimization gleaned from hundreds of lectures given by anti-aging physicians and supported by research presented in medical journals. This book focuses on how to lose toxic belly fat and regain metabolic health by correcting the sick metabolism associated with toxic belly fat.

Book One: "Secrets about Bioidentical Hormones to Lose Fat and Prevent Cancer, Heart Disease, Menopause, and Andropause by Optimizing Adrenals, Thyroid, Estrogen, Progesterone, Testosterone, and Growth Hormone!" Feel great, look great, lose weight, and have better sex! Discover groundbreaking scientific secrets about bioidentical hormones unknown to most people, including most physicians. Use the guidance of hundreds of anti-aging physicians and researchers to minimize and reverse aging. Learn how hormonal and metabolic disturbances make you sick and fat. Women may change their life and feel young again using the Wiley protocol to mimic the cyclic monthly hormones of a healthy 20-year old. Understand imbalances in insulin, adrenal hormones, thyroid hormones, growth hormone, and sex hormones. Find out how hormones become deficient and unbalanced, especially during menopause and andropause. Replace missing hormones AND minimize your cancer risk. Use this book to work with a forward-thinking, knowledgeable physician in your area who will prescribe ALL of the bioidentical hormones that you need in the dosages and rhythms needed.

No other book available presents hormonal optimization in such a comprehensive and integrated manner.

Book Two: "Bioidentical Hormones Made Easy!" Learn about bioidentical hormone replacement therapy (BHRT) in a quick and easy book. Learn about the history of hormone replacement therapy (HRT) and discover how all HRT became feared, even bioidentical hormones. Learn how to find a doctor who will help you and not hurt you. Explore all of your BHRT options, learning how to replace your hormones safely, so that you can prevent heart disease, cancer, and all other diseases of aging.

Book Three: "Secrets About Growth Hormone to Build Muscle, Increase Bone Density, and Burn Body Fat!" GROWTH HORMONE (GH) IS A HOT TOPIC. It seems that all of the movie stars, celebrities, and body-builders are taking it, and they look fantastic. Baby boomers interested in anti-aging are taking it and saying that it keeps them young. But you may have heard that it is expensive... and dangerous. So what's the story? What are your options? Do you need it? Should you take it? How do you use it? Can you afford it? How can you raise GH naturally? We will see how GH levels drop as we get older, when to intervene, and what treatment options are available to optimize health. Carefully read this book before making any decisions about using GH supplements. This book could save you from an early death, either from using risky supplements, or from not using them when you need them. You will learn how to determine if you need GH replacement. You will find out how to get tested and what tests you will need. You will learn what options you have for GH replacement, risks, side effects, and affordability.

Book Four: "Fat Loss Secrets that Really Work--Balance Your Hormones: Insulin, Estrogen, Progesterone, Testosterone, Thyroid, Cortisol, and DHEA!" Read this book and learn the secrets that will enable you to regain your health, look great, feel great, lose weight, and have better sex! Discover how everyone can be permanently successful with fat loss without resorting to one of the latest diet fads. Popular weight-loss methods and diets do not work long-term and may be dangerous to your health when followed for any length of time. The problem is that none of these popular weight-loss methods consider your hormones. Most overweight people have unbalanced hormones, more so if they have been dieting on and off for years and years. Find out exactly how to correct the hormonal problems that prevent you from losing fat, especially belly fat, and how to normalize your weight for the rest of your life.

Book Five: "Secrets about the HCG Diet! Treatment Guide, Controversy, Benefits, Risks, Side Effects, and Contraindications." Find out the pros and cons of using the hCG protocol to lose weight. Read this unbiased information to learn the benefits, the warnings, the off-label usage, the contradictions, the side-effects, and the contraindications (health conditions for which the hCG protocol could be harmful). Discover the answers to: What is hCG? How does hCG work? How is it used in a program to lose weight? What are its other uses? What treatment modalities work most effectively? What are the specifics of the hCG diet protocol? What are the side effects? How can I do the diet safely? What else do I need to know to take the weight off and keep it off? This book includes a detailed guide to follow the hCG protocol. Learn how to prepare yourself to do this powerful weight-loss protocol safely, taking every possible precaution to avoid problems.

All of these books may be purchased in either print or downloadable versions at: http://www.lulu.com/spotlight/treewise

Table of Contents

INTRODUCTION 6

Step I. LEARN ABOUT SICK METABOLISM. 9
  A. SICK METABOLISM FROM TOXICITY. 9
    1. Escalating environmental toxicity. *10*
    2. Increasing toxicity = increasing disease. *13*
    3. Metals and chemicals harm us. *14*
    4. Toxins damage cells. *15*
    5. Toxins damage mitochondria. *15*
    6. Heavy metals = health problems. *16*
    7. Chemicals make us sick. *18*
  B. SICK METABOLISM FROM INFECTIOUS DISEASE. 22
    1. Bacterial infections are often present. *23*
    2. Viral infections are increasing. *23*
    3. Parasites are often undiagnosed. *24*
    4. Leaky gut leads to food allergies. *24*
    5. Undiagnosed yeast infections are common. *25*
  C. SICK METABOLISM FROM HORMONAL IMBALANCE. 25
    1. Toxic belly fat = insulin resistance. *25*
    2. Adrenal dysfunction and cortisol. *26*
    3. DHEA is anabolic and balances cortisol. *27*
    4. Improve thyroid function. *28*
    5. Leptin and ghrelin backfire. *29*
    6. Progesterone in females. *30*
    7. Estrogen in females. *30*
    8. Testosterone in females. *31*
    9. Testosterone in males. *31*
    10. Estrogen in males. *31*
    11. HGH declines with age. *31*
    12. Estrogen metabolism & cancer. *32*
    13. Neurotransmitter imbalances. *32*

Step II. GET STATE-OF-THE-ART TESTING. 33
  A. TEST FOR TOXICITY. 35
    1. Test oxidative damage and screen for toxicity. *35*
    2. Test for heavy metal toxicity. *36*
    3. Test for specific chemical toxins. *37*
  B. SCREEN FOR INFECTIOUS DISEASE OF THE G.I. TRACT. 38
    1. Test for bacterial infections. *38*
    2. Test for viruses. *38*
    3. Test for parasites. *39*
    4. Test for yeast. *40*
    5. Test for leaky gut. *40*
  C. TEST HORMONES. 40
    1. Adrenal health testing. *40*
    2. Insulin resistance testing. *41*
    3. Thyroid health testing. *41*
    4. Female sex hormone testing. *41*
    5. Male sex hormone testing. *42*
    6. Human Growth Hormone testing. *42*
    7. Estrogen metabolism testing. *42*

D. CHECK MARKERS FOR INFLAMMATION...............................43
E. CHECK NEUROTRANSMITTER LEVELS...............................43

Step III. INDIVIDUALIZE TREATMENT PLANS. **44**
A. TREAT TOXICITY. 44
    1. Don't take in the poisons....*45*
    2. Open elimination channels. *49*
    3. Eliminate heavy metals and chemicals..............................*54*
    4. Increase alkalinity....*56*
    5. Avoid EMR....*56*
    6. Continue to detox for life. *56*
B. TREAT INFECTIOUS DISEASE...57
    1. Boost immunity. *58*
    2. Treat bacterial infections...*59*
    3. Treat viral infections. *59*
    4. Treat parasites...*59*
    5. Treat leaky gut. *60*
    6. Treat heartburn....*60*
    7. Treat yeast. *61*
    8. Treat dysbiosis....*61*
C. TREAT HORMONAL DYSFUNCTION......................................61
    1. Treat insulin resistance....*61*
    2. Treat adrenal dysfunction. *64*
    3. Treat thyroid dysfunction. *66*
    4. Bioidentical Hormone Replacement Therapy (BHRT). *67*
    5. Women: replace sex hormones. *67*
    6. Treat andropause...*69*
    7. Correct faulty estrogen metabolism..................................*71*
    8. Optimize Human Growth Hormone. *72*
    9. Restore leptin sensitivity...*72*
    10. Restore ghrelin sensitivity....*72*
D. TREAT INFLAMMATION. 72
E. TREAT MITOCHONDRIAL DYSFUNCTION. 73
F. REPAIR CELL DAMAGE. 73
G. OPTIMIZE NEUROTRANSMITTER LEVELS.............................74
    1. Serotonin—master neurotransmitter. *75*
    2. Acetylcholine....*76*
    3. Noradrenaline. *76*
    4. Dopamine. *76*
    5. GABA. *77*

IMPLEMENT THE SECRET ACTION PLAN! **78**

REFERENCES...**79**

INDEX **91**

INTRODUCTION

Toxic BELLY FAT IS THE WORST KIND OF FAT.

Toxic belly fat is a parasite that preserves itself at the expense of its host – YOU. At a certain point, toxic belly fat takes on a life of its own, fighting to preserve itself.

Toxic Belly Fat (TBF) is the fat that has concentrated around the abdomen and chest. The *classic* definition of toxic belly fat is the fat that has collected in the middle of your body, totally sparing the extremities. Most of the fat collects in the abdominal area. The lack of fat in the arms and legs, especially in the legs, makes it easy to spot toxic belly fat in people who don't have excess fat on other parts of their bodies. People with excess fat on other parts of their body may also have toxic belly fat. You may have a lot of fat on your hips and still have toxic belly fat. You may be fat all over and still have toxic belly fat.

Toxic belly fat produces hormones that keep you hungry, never let you feel satisfied, and make you continue to gain weight. Toxic belly fat acts avidly to prevent weight loss. The toxic fat that deposits itself in the abdominal area and chest acts differently from the fat all over the rest of the body. Toxic belly fat *makes* hormones. Belly fat, more than overall body fat, is strongly linked with insulin resistance, hyperandrogenism in women (too many male hormones), diabetes, hypertension (high blood pressure), and hyperlipidemia (abnormally high lipids).[1]

Hormones and chemicals produced by toxic belly fat keep us fat and diabetic.[2] Belly fat is a highly-active endocrine (hormone-producing) and inflammatory organ that produces a vast array of hormones and chemicals that affect metabolism.[3] The hormones and chemicals produced by belly fat create insulin resistance and other pathological reactions. As belly fat accumulates, we begin to see dyslipidemia (abnormal fats in the blood), characterized by high circulating triglycerides, low HDL (good cholesterol), and accelerated development of atherosclerosis (hardening of the arteries). It is a vicious cycle that is hard to break if you don't know how.

Insulin resistance underlies the basic formation of toxic belly fat, and toxic belly fat perpetuates insulin resistance. As insulin resistance increases in response to the hormones and chemicals produced by belly fat, there is a decreased ability of insulin to shut off glucose release from the liver and to move glucose into muscle, where it could be burned for energy. This leads to high blood sugar and the development of metabolic syndrome and diabetes.

Most Americans have toxic belly fat. Toxic belly fat is epidemic because our dietary habits and lack of exercise have created insulin resistance, and we all live in a polluted world. Some people have more toxic belly fat than others, because their diet is more unregulated, and they have a greater toxic burden. Toxic belly fat is caused by the constant and steady ingestion of dead processed food, high glycemic loads of carbohydrates, toxic heavy metals, pesticides, herbicides, and other toxins.

Toxins make belly fat, and belly fat makes us more toxic. It is an ever-worsening downward spiral. It works like this:
(1) As we take in toxins or create toxins through super-saturating our body with sugar from high-glycemic loads (processed sugar and carbohydrates), the toxins create sick metabolism and insulin resistance, which form belly fat.
(2) As belly fat forms, it produces more toxins and sickens metabolism even more.
(3) All of this toxicity accumulates in the tissues, and health deteriorates.

In order to escape from this insidious downward spiral, follow the lifestyle and dietary recommendations given in this book. They are based on sound principles of physiology and are designed to free you from disease. Implementing the advice given in this book will greatly improve *anyone's* health, no matter how much fat they have accumulated.

MANY CURRENT DIETARY RECOMMENDATIONS OF TRUSTED AUTHORITIES ARE COUNTER-PRODUCTIVE IN THE LONG RUN.[4]

The dietary recommendations of many traditional medical practitioners are based on the USDA Food Pyramid. Unfortunately, the food pyramid has ignored the importance of avoiding highly-processed refined foods and has not advocated eating LIVE foods. The food pyramid also has neglected to advise us to avoid preservatives, chemicals, hormones, and other toxins in our food and to stay away from the high-glycemic foods that create insulin resistance.

The food pyramid was developed in an attempt to avert the epidemic of heart disease. As evidenced by the increasing obesity and disease in our society, the food pyramid has failed to reduce heart disease and has led to worsening of many health problems. The food pyramid's emphasis on eating more carbohydrates and fewer fats contributes to the epidemic of insulin resistance, metabolic syndrome, and type 2 diabetes.

With low-fat diets, the body lacks the fats necessary for hormone production, building healthy cells, and healthy metabolism. Inadequate high-quality fats and excessive high-glycemic loads ruin health and metabolism. The high-carbohydrate loads associated with low-fat diets produce insulin resistance and sick metabolism. High-quality fats are needed to form hormones. Plenty of high-quality protein is needed to form the building blocks of every tissue in the body. When high-quality proteins and fats are removed from the diet, health havoc is the ultimate result.

With high-fat, low-carbohydrate diets, after six months to a year or two, hormones and neurotransmitters become imbalanced. Then people return to carbohydrates, often craving sweets to raise serotonin. Serotonin is the master neurotransmitter that controls mood and hormones. Restricting carbohydrates drops serotonin. Without serotonin, the hormones that control metabolism and weight become impaired.

TARGETING THE PATHOPHYSIOLOGY OF TOXIC BELLY FAT WILL RETURN YOU TO HEALTH, INSULIN SENSITIVITY, AND WEIGHT NORMALIZATION. Understanding the underlying pathology of toxic belly fat is critical if you want to overcome this common disease of modern life.

It is a journey, not a destination. The only answer to regaining health and elimination of toxic belly fat is to eat correctly (live, healthy foods, not dead processed foods), to exercise, to identify and remove poisonous toxins, to identify and overcome all infections (even those that are silent), and to identify hormonal imbalances and correct them.

It took many years to impair your metabolism with improper diet and taking in toxicity. If you want to heal your sick metabolism and lose the toxic belly fat for good, you must have patience. You must follow the secret action plan and work with your physician. So let's begin the journey right away.

READ THIS BOOK:

(1) Discover how damaged metabolism caused by toxins, infections, and abnormal and/or inadequate hormones creates toxic belly fat (TBF).

(2) Find out how to get the relatively unknown state-of-the-art medical tests that will reveal hidden toxicities, infections, and hormonal imbalances. This book extensively details *all* of the testing that you will need to get so that your physician can accurately diagnose and treat you. The testing guide may be used by both you and your physician to make sure that you are getting each and every specialty test that is required to uncover all of the causes of *your* sick metabolism.

(3) Under your doctor's supervision, tailor the treatment suggestions to remove the causes of *your* sick metabolism that have been identified by the results of *your* state-of-the-art testing.

ELIMINATE THE THREE MAJOR CAUSES OF SICK METABOLISM THAT CAUSE TOXIC BELLY FAT:

(1) Remove the toxins. The staggering amount of environmental pollution that has contaminated our planet has also polluted each and every one of us.[5] Get the state-of-the art medical testing that is recommended in this book to identify exactly which toxins are present in *your* tissues and to determine the extent of the damage that they have caused in *your* body.[6] Under your physician's guidance, follow the step-by-step guide to safely remove the toxins that have been pinpointed in *your* test results. After lowering your toxic burden, your own hormones and any supplemental bioidentical hormones that you are taking will become more effective.

(2) Eradicate infection. Learn how to overcome any chronic smoldering infection(s) that may have been eating away at you for years. Overcome bacterial, viral, parasitic, and yeast infections in your gut, your mouth, your throat, your sinuses, your respiratory tract, and your skin. Understand how a wide range of viruses, including stealth viruses and genetically-engineered strains, are attacking many of us. Discover how parasites are often undiagnosed and lead to many health problems, especially leaky gut. Learn where to get state-of-the art medical testing to find out exactly what infections are dragging *you* down. After identifying *your* infections, work with your physician to implement the treatment plan to completely eradicate each and every infection.

(3) Optimize your hormones. Discover how to balance the hormones that control your appetite, your mood, and your weight. Learn how to get the right state-of-the-art medical tests to determine *your own* specific hormone imbalances in insulin, cortisol, DHEA, thyroid, leptin, ghrelin, estrogen, progesterone, testosterone, and growth hormone. Recognize neurotransmitter imbalances and measure the degree of inflammation. Identify faulty estrogen metabolism, which, if not corrected, may increase the risk of cancer of the reproductive organs in both men and women. After ascertaining hormonal, neurotransmitter, inflammation, and estrogen metabolism status, under your physician's supervision, follow the treatment plan for lifestyle changes, diet, and bioidentical hormone replacement (BHRT) to heal each imbalance.

READ THIS BOOK AND DISCOVER A SECRET ACTION PLAN to heal your sick metabolism, lose toxic belly fat, and overcome chronic disease.
This secret action plan was formulated from decades of clinical experience, advice from the leading experts in anti-aging, and research studies published in medical journals. Implement the secret action plan with your physician, and your attempts to lose weight will finally be fruitful!

YOUR SECRET ACTION PLAN HAS THREE STEPS:

Step I: Educate yourself about the sick metabolism that underlies toxic belly fat.

Step II: Find out exactly how your metabolism has become sick using very specialized state-of-the-art medical tests. Get the most advanced anti-aging testing available in the world.

Step III: Individualize the detailed treatment plans. Use your state-of-the-art medical testing results to educate yourself and assist your physician in diagnosing and treating *your* health problems. Then you will lose that stubborn toxic belly fat and reverse and eliminate chronic disease. You will look great, feel great, lose weight, and have better sex!

Step I. LEARN ABOUT SICK METABOLISM.

Eliminate THE THREE MAJOR CAUSES OF SICK METABOLISM THAT CAUSE TOXIC BELLY FAT:

A. REMOVE THE TOXINS. Sick metabolism is caused by belly fat that has been poisoned with toxicity. Belly fat causes toxicity, and toxicity causes belly fat. Read on and learn to break this vicious cycle.

B. ERADICATE INFECTION. Chronic infections add to the vicious cycle of inflammation and toxic belly fat production. Infections prevent you from losing toxic belly fat. Read on and learn how to any conquer smoldering infection(s) that may have been eating away at you for years, even infections that have minimal or no symptoms.

C. OPTIMIZE YOUR HORMONES. Hormonal imbalance causes sick metabolism. Belly fat *produces* chemicals and hormones that determine your weight and level of health. Hormones that control hunger and satiety can backfire, causing you to get fatter. As hormone levels change in menopause and andropause, you may get even fatter. Read on and learn how to control the hormones that make toxic belly fat.

A. SICK METABOLISM FROM TOXICITY.

*T*OXICITY IS AN OFTEN-OVERLOOKED FACTOR *that is responsible for the destruction of our health.* Toxins include heavy metals, infectious disease, foreign chemicals, and products of abnormal metabolism.

TOXINS HARM US IN MANY WAYS:

- *Toxins make us fat.*[7] [8] [9] The chemical and heavy metal toxins, which were unknown to our ancestors, accumulate in the fat around our abdomen and chest creating a body burden.[10] Toxins may prevent every other weight-loss and health strategy from working by impairing metabolism.[11]
- *Toxins cause the aches and pains* that we associate with aging.
- *The immune system becomes depressed or hyperactive.*[12]
- *Auto-immune disorders become more likely.* Examples of auto-immune disorders include osteo-arthritis, allergies, lupus, and M.S.
- *Toxins block the proper functioning of the body, especially hormonal function.*[13] You cannot efficiently use your own hormones or even supplemental bioidentical hormones when toxins are present in the body. Some act as hormone mimickers and bind the receptor site. Other toxins may disrupt the cell membrane (where the receptor sites are located) or even cause the loss of the receptor sites.

There are over 80,000 chemicals on our planet that were not present one hundred years ago. Over 80,000 chemicals have been approved for use by the U.S. Environmental Protection Agency for use in the USA.[14]

When you eat a pesticide on your food or breathe it in after it has been sprayed, you are getting the same neurotoxic poison that is designed to kill insects. Most of these poisons are highly fat-soluble and are particularly dangerous and difficult to remove when ingested.

Fat-soluble toxins are soluble in the body's fat stores. If the fat is lost, the toxins are released, and if the body is not prepared to excrete them, they are redistributed to the remaining fat stores, matrix, and vital organs.

Our bodies lock up the toxins in the matrix to protect us. This is a very new concept, unheard of by most people. You probably will not see it anywhere else until it catches on. Right now it is our little secret.

The organs of elimination can only process a small amount of poison at a time. When you have ingested more than just a tiny bit of poison, your body must protect its vulnerable organs (like the brain, heart, liver, and kidneys) from the damaging effects that would occur if the poison were allowed to roam free in the bloodstream.

Your body is like the government that buries nuclear waste in underground storage facilities far, far away from big cities . . . until it can figure out what to do with it. Your body buries the poison in the space that separates the capillaries (tiny blood vessels) from the cells, far, far away from vital organs . . . until it can figure out what to do with it.

This poison-holding space is called the extracellular matrix. The matrix space contains a complex mixture of proteins and sugars, called proteoglycans. These proteoglycans have multiple binding sites that are designed to trap and bind toxins in the body. This is the body's way of sequestering toxins from deposition in the vital organs, especially in the brain and kidneys. Toxins accumulate in the matrix around the cells. It may only be one part per billion or one part per million, but they don't leave.[15] The toxins accumulate over months and years and lifetimes (being passed from mother to child).

The matrix becomes a toxic swamp, and toxic belly fat builds up. The nutrients that must get from the capillary bed to nourish the cells have to diffuse across the toxic swamp, and metabolic products must get back through this toxic swamp to be carried away by the organs of elimination. Metabolism slows down and diseases develop. The metabolism becomes sick.

1. Escalating environmental toxicity.

The air that we breathe, the water that we drink, and the food that we eat, are all contaminated with massive amounts of heavy metals, pesticides, herbicides, plastic residues, and many other chemicals. Many billions of pounds of toxic waste, including pesticides and herbicides, are released into the water and air of the United States in a year. In the state of Texas alone, over three billion pounds of toxic waste were disposed of in the year 2010. These wastes went into the air, water, and ground. These only included wastes that were reported to the Environmental Protection Agency (EPA). Who knows what and how much unreported toxicity went into the environment? We are all breathing toxic waste, drinking toxic waste, and eating toxic waste in massive amounts.

The magnetic field in which we live is polluted with microwave radiation and other disturbing frequencies coming from cell phones, wireless devices, cell phone towers, antennas, "smart" electric meters, radio frequency devices placed in our pets, alternating electric currents, and high-voltage power lines.

Our air is contaminated.

Heavy metals and chemicals are being sprayed into the air that we breathe. Over 87,000 jet airplanes fly back and forth over the United States every day. Just as lead was added to gasoline in the late 1920's to keep cars from backfiring, heavy metals are added to jet fuel to keep jets flying smoothly.

We are constantly breathing in hydrocarbons from auto emissions, as well. Pesticides and herbicides are being sprayed into the air like there is no tomorrow.[16] And indeed, there may be no tomorrow for those of us who don't take steps to eliminate these poisons from our bodies. There may be no tomorrow for our children either, as environmentally-caused cancer steals their lives from them at an ever-increasing rate.[17]

Our water is contaminated.

The poisons being sprayed into the air and applied to the earth are getting into the water. Before we drink the water, even more chemicals are added. In

1904, they began adding chlorine to the water to reduce bacteria. Within twenty years, **cardiovascular disease** had increased dramatically. Many people believe that this was a direct result of tap water chlorination. Drinking chlorinated water may also cause **poor digestion**, because chlorine kills the bacteria in your gut, causing dysbiosis (imbalanced gut flora).

Water chlorination has also been implicated in bladder and rectal **cancer**.[18] [19] [20] If you seriously considered all of the cases of all kinds of cancer directly related to drinking tap water, you would not drink it (unless you were suicidal). You wouldn't swim in it either.

If you drink tap water, you are getting quite an array of chemicals, including prescription drugs, which add up in your body to produce **ill health**. As more and more chemicals are added, the negative effects increase exponentially. The interaction of all of these chemicals makes the toxic soup of tap water a very dangerous health hazard.

There is very little water available on the planet that has not been polluted. Even if you have a well or drink from a pristine stream, the water often contains dangerous amounts of heavy metals and chemicals or infectious disease, like giardia (a parasite). The pollutants leech into the water from contaminated soil and air.

Our soil and food are contaminated.

Eating food is how we get a lot of the toxicity in our bodies, a problem unknown to our ancestors, even a hundred years ago. The poisons that are being sprayed into the air and added to the water are taken up by the plants and animals that we eat. Food producers deliberately add many toxic chemicals to the soil and onto the plants that we eat as herbicides to kill weeds and pesticides to kill bugs. Animal feed is polluted with a wide variety of hormones, drugs, and other toxins. Our dairy, meat, fish, and chicken are contaminated with pesticides, herbicides, heavy metals, and other chemicals, which then concentrate in our tissues when we consume them.

Even if you eat organic food, you cannot completely escape metals, herbicides and pesticides. Even organic food may contain heavy metals that cause those who eat it to become heavy-metal toxic. Some of the chemicals that have been approved for use on organic farms are now being associated with cancer. "Rotenone" is a pesticide primarily used by organic farmers. But just like its more toxic counterparts, this "organic" pesticide knocks out mitochondrial function, destroying the ability of cells to make energy. Rotenone ingestion also leads to neurological damage.[21]

Beef cattle in the U.S. are given hormones to fatten them up. Diethylstilbestrol (DES) that was used in the past proved to be so carcinogenic that it was finally banned. But U.S. cattle and poultry are still routinely given hormones and dosed with antibiotics, even if they are healthy.[22] Because of health risks to humans from eating beef that comes from cattle given hormones, all hormone-dosed meat is banned in Canada and the European Union. U.S. beef is not allowed to be imported into those countries.

Caged poultry and farm-raised fish are raised in an extremely toxic environment,[23] *given drugs, and fed unnatural food.*[24] [25] It is cruel to the animals. Chicken feed is loaded with arsenic to fatten the chickens.[26] Arsenic may cause cancer,[27] dementia, and neurological problems in the people who eat the chickens.[28] Farm-raised salmon are raised in overcrowded conditions, increasing risk of infection and disease. Farm-raised salmon are not fed their normal diet of krill with its high Omega-3 concentrations.[29] They are fed dried food pellets that often are contaminated with antibiotics and cancer-causing PCBs, dioxins, and flame retardants.[30] Farm-raised salmon is white, because these fish don't eat the carotenoids that give wild salmon their pink color. Canthaxanthin pigment is added to make it look palatable. Consuming canthaxanthin pigment causes retinal damage[31] and is banned in Great Britain.

Even the fish that roam freely in the sea are contaminated with mercury. The ocean is becoming more and more polluted with this insidious metal that manufacturers dump into our air and waters. Bigger fish pose more of a problem because they eat the little fish and the mercury becomes more concentrated in their tissues.[32]

Dairy cattle in the U.S. are given bovine growth hormone (BGH) to increase milk production. Researchers have concluded that, "Prostate and breast cancer patients should be cautioned about the possible promotional effects of commercial dairy products and their substitutes."[33]

Genetic modification (GMO) is the latest insult to our food. The process of genetic modification involves inserting bacteria and viruses into the DNA inside the nucleus of the plant cell. In the United States, foods are not labeled as GMO (Genetically Modified Organisms). But in Europe, they must be labeled.[34] [35] Giant corporations have taken over the seed supply through patents and litigation against any farmers who do not go along with their agenda to make sure that the major crops grown in the United States are all genetically-modified. These GMO crops make huge profits for the corporations. GMO seeds have been developed that produce plants that can resist the herbicide produced by the corporation. Thus they can spray herbicide on the crops without killing the crops.

The FDA has now approved Roundup-resistant beets. The only reason to develop GMO Roundup-resistant beets is to allow this herbicide to be heavily sprayed on the beets.

Corporations profit:
    (1) From the sale of the herbicide.
    (2) From the sale of the GMO crops.

Consumers suffer:
    (1) From the herbicide entering their bodies.
    (2) From the negative effects of eating genetically-modified food.

Studies testing the safety of GMO foods are sparse from U.S. researchers, but researchers in Europe have voiced their concern. Researchers in the Netherlands have said, "The intensified use of viruses and their genetically modified variants as viral gene transfer vectors for biomedical research, experimental gene therapy and for live-vector vaccines is a cause for concern."[36] Researchers in Copenhagen stated, "The introduction of novel proteins into foods carries a risk of eliciting allergic reactions in individuals sensitive to the introduced protein and a risk of sensitizing susceptible individuals."[37] A researcher in Rome summarizes the problem, "Genetic engineering poses innovative ethical and social concerns, as well as serious challenges to the environment, human health, animal welfare, and the future of agriculture."[38]

We don't even know how bad the problem really is. By altering our food supply at the genetic level we may be harming unborn children for generations to come (assuming that people don't become totally sterile and unable to bear children).[39]

The most common GMO foods in this country today are beets, canola, soybeans, cotton, and corn. Even crops that are not genetically-modified will all eventually be contaminated with seed from the GMO crops and will have negative health effects. Wheat is the next target for massive GMO contamination.

Our magnetic field is contaminated.

Before the advent of electricity, the major magnetic field we knew was that of the earth. The human body naturally resonates with the low magnetic field from the earth. The earth's field is a very low direct current.

Now we are living in an ocean of electromagnetic radiation that was unknown to mankind a hundred years ago. It is coming from the alternating currents in our homes and buildings, cell phones, microwaves, and wireless devices. As the years go by, the forms and levels of electromagnetic radiation have increased exponentially. Electromagnetic radiation may cause sleeplessness, weight gain and general fatigue. It is also associated with cancer.[40]

The alternating current (AC) wires in our homes are a disturbing frequency for our bodies. The alternating currents that surround us in our home change direction sixty times per second, creating an oscillating magnetic field. This is in sharp contrast to the magnetic field of the earth that only flows in one direction. If you live near a high-voltage power line, the oscillating magnetic field is much stronger. There have been studies showing a connection between childhood leukemia and living near these high-voltage power lines.[41] Electromagnetic radiation is highest within 300 feet of these high-voltage lines.

Cell phones are associated with brain cancer.[42] The brain tumors are found in the right side of the brain in people who hold their cell phones up to the right side of their head and on the left side of the brain in people who hold their cell phones up to the left side of their head.

Cell phones increase our risk of disease from exposure to all of the heavy metals and chemicals in our environment. Researchers have found that the use of cell phones disrupts the integrity of the blood brain barrier.[43] When the integrity of the blood brain barrier has been breached, dangerous chemicals can cross unimpeded into the brain.

We are bombarded by microwave radiation. We have over a hundred thousand cell phone towers and two million antennas in the United States, and they are increasing in number every day. Cell phone towers emit microwave radiation. Microwave radiation excites electrons and heats them up. D.O. Carpenter summarizes the problem, "Standards are set at levels designed to avoid tissue heating, in spite of convincing evidence of adverse biological effects at intensities too low to cause significant heating."[44]

Microwave radiation excites your electrons and wakes you up. When you are sleeping, you are being exposed to the microwave radiation from cell phone calls and computer signals which are being bounced off of the cell phone towers. The body interprets this excitation much as if the sun had come up. Your body thinks it is time to get up, even if is really the middle of the night. The EMR (electrosmog) coming from the wireless technology that everyone else is using while you are sleeping has a similar effect on your brain as turning on the light in your bedroom. Your brain is being signaled to wake up.

RFID transmitters are the latest insult. These are chips that they put into pets to locate them when they get lost. There have been anecdotal reports that within a few years of insertion, pets with these chips develop tumors in the areas where the chips were inserted. They are talking about putting them into people.

"Smart meters" are devices that are now being installed on electric meters everywhere. They send a signal out about once an hour that goes to a cell phone tower. If you are waking up every hour, this may be connected.

The role of microwave radiation in our health decline is not being officially recognized. People have become too comfortable with the technology to seek regulation for industries that use wireless technology. Instead of being warned of the deleterious effects of microwave radiation on our health, we have been lulled into a false sense of security. The danger of microwave radiation, especially on those who live in cities, is being ignored.

2. Increasing toxicity = increasing disease.

People were not always this toxic. The remains of mummies from thousands of years ago have no traces of cancer, even in those who died of advanced age.[45] [46] Cancer became common only after the beginnings of the industrial revolution.

Now our tissues have become permeated with heavy metals and other toxic chemicals that lead to cancer and other degenerative diseases.[47] We *all* have this problem, and it is getting worse all the time. Along with inadequate nutrition, toxicity may be blamed for our worldwide epidemics of obesity, immune disorders, cancer, heart disease, neurological disorders, and other illness.

The problem exists all over the world. Environmental policies are totally absent or inadequate to prevent the contamination. Heavy metals go into the jet stream and drop down onto us. Herbicides and pesticides permeate the air and spread quickly over the entire globe every day. The EPA, the CDC, the FDA, and state health departments are all monitoring our exposure to these cell-damaging substances. But nobody is doing very much to *prevent* environmental contamination.

Today, the environment plays a much larger role in causing the development of cancer and chronic degenerative disease than most people realize.[48] Inherited genetic factors play a minor role in most cancer expression.[49] Researchers at M.D. Anderson Cancer Center at the University of Texas have concluded that "only 5–10% of all cancer cases can be attributed to genetic defects, whereas the remaining 90–95% of all cancer cases stem from environment and lifestyle."[50] Even if you don't have any genetic tendency toward developing cancer, xenoestrogens from the environment in the form of heavy metals, pesticides, plastics, cosmetics, perfumes, and other chemicals act as "bad" estrogens, adding to your risk of getting cancer, particularly endometrial, ovarian, and breast cancer in women[51] [52] and prostate cancer in men.[53] [54]

Each generation is more toxic than the generation before. Toxins are passed from mother to unborn child in the placenta.[55] As heavy metal levels rise, the levels of heavy metals in breast milk also rises.[56] [57] Many toxins are present in baby formula, as well.[58]

As these toxins are passed from mother to child, toxicity in the tissues of each succeeding generation increases dramatically. As the chemicals in our environment become more and more ubiquitous, children of each successive generation are born with greater and greater toxic loads. Some experts suspect that the autism epidemic may have been triggered by the faulty dietary habits and toxic burden passed on to these children by their mothers and grandmothers.

Cancer rates are increasing dramatically. Cancer is the number one disease killing U.S. children aged 1-15.[59] In recent years, cancer rates have soared all over the world. Worldwide breast cancer incidence increased from about 641,000 cases in 1980 to about 1,643,000 cases in 2010. That is an annual rate of increase of 3.1%![60]

3. Metals and chemicals harm us.

Heavy metals and chemicals are all foreign substances that harm the body. Toxicity affects everyone, everywhere.[61] Simple things like getting a new car or painting your walls may seriously harm your health.[62]

Whether it is a heavy metal or an organochemical, toxins dramatically harm us by blocking all of the proper functions of the body's organs. These are serious toxins that contribute to the cause of Parkinson's and other neurological disorders,[63] cancer,[64] heart disease,[65] atherosclerosis,[66] and thyroid problems.[67] Heavy metals are a big problem for the bones. Lead, aluminum, and other heavy metals will displace the calcium in the bones.

Toxins interfere with hormonal balance (especially xenotoxins). Heavy metals and chemicals can damage the hormone receptors on the cell walls. Xenotoxins are similar to the hormones of the body and can bind to the receptor and displace the body's hormones. Xenoestrogens are prevalent in toxic metals and in the phthalates from plastics, pesticides, and herbicides.

Toxins block insulin from coming into the cells, causing insulin resistance. We become insulin-resistant when our insulin receptors aren't working right. The insulin receptors don't work right when toxins are blocking the insulin from coming into the cells. These toxins are metabolic interrupters. They cause obesity or sicken the metabolism so badly that weight loss occurs.

Multiple metals and chemical toxins, which we all have, compound the danger. Everyone's test results show multiple heavy metals and chemical toxins. The mix of multiple toxic metals and chemicals produces toxic effects greater than the sum of the parts.

Most physicians know that high levels of individual metals cause problems. Acute heavy metal poisoning (especially lead poisoning in children) is treated seriously by most physicians.

But few traditional physicians are aware of the harmful effects of the low levels of multiple heavy metals. Nor do they understand how these metals react in the presence of low levels of multiple chemical toxins. Anti-aging physicians understand the danger of low to moderate levels of multiple metals and chemical toxins.

4. Toxins damage cells.

Toxins damage the cell membrane through a process called oxidative stress.[68] Oxidative stress involves burning the cell membrane by free radicals.[69] Cells communicate with each other through the cell membranes. When cell membranes are injured, the cells of the tissue and the tissues of the organs can't work properly. Toxins disrupt the health of every cell, every tissue, and every organ by damaging cell membranes.

The cell membrane has two layers of phospholipids that are very susceptible to being burned by the free radicals generated by heavy metals and other toxins.[70] These free radicals dissolve the cell membranes. The cells develop cracks and burned spots which need to be repaired if they are ever going to work right again. Unless the cell membranes are repaired, vitamins or nutrients from healthy food cannot get into the cells. Heavy metals, particularly lead, prevent cell membrane repair.[71]

5. Toxins damage mitochondria.

One major reason for the disruption to our health caused by toxins is the damage caused to the mitochondria.[72] Mitochondria are the organelles inside all of our cells that make energy. They are the powerhouses of the cells. Ten per cent of the body weight is made up of mitochondria.

Some of the substances that harm mitochondrial function are all very, very common compounds that are in all of us. Once in the mitochondria, toxins cause all kinds of havoc. Toxins compromise our mitochondrial function in multiple ways and then prevent us from clearing out toxins. It's an ugly cycle that disrupts health.

Mitochondrial damage may come from a depletion of glutathione. The depletion of glutathione in the inner mitochondrial membrane is thought to lead to the impermeability of the membrane so that protons can't be pumped to make ATP (energy). It increases reactive oxygen species (free radicals). And of course, it causes cell apoptosis, or cell death.[73]

When the toxins damage our mitochondria, we get sick and tired. The wide variety of chronic illness that is caused by toxins stems from their ability to hinder mitochondrial function. People who have chronic fatigue and fibromyalgia usually have mitochondrial dysfunction or loss of mitochondria. Mitochondrial mutations are found in many cancers.

Common diseases associated with mitochondrial dysfunction include:
- Diabetes (a current epidemic).
- Insulin resistance (a current epidemic, especially with children).
- Obesity (a current epidemic).
- Hepatic steatosis (fatty liver).
- Cancer.
- Chronic fatigue.
- Chronic neurologic problems.
- Cardiac myopathy (muscular weakness of the heart).
- Parkinson's.[74]

Fatigue is the most common complaint of people who have been exposed to environmental toxins. When the powerhouses of the cells aren't working well, we get tired. When our mitochondria aren't working well, we cannot produce the energy that we need to feel vibrant and healthy. When toxins begin to disrupt the healthy function of the mitochondria, our health deteriorates. This deterioration is often referred to as aging.

With all of the toxicity in our environment damaging our mitochondria, is it any wonder why so many of us are so tired? Ask any doctor and you will get the same answer. Most of their patients present with fatigue as one of their top five complaints.

When mitochondrial function is suppressed by toxins, it damages (1) the immune system, (2) the neurologic system, and (3) the endocrine system.[75] The damage usually begins in one of these systems and eventually moves on to the other systems.

(1) If the damage involves the immune system, people develop allergies and asthma, two conditions that are becoming more and more common all over the globe. Chemical sensitivity may appear, as well. Auto-immune conditions stem from toxic damage to the immune system. The immune system is constantly removing cancerous cells, and impairment of the immune system increases cancer rates.

(2) When the toxins damage the neurologic system, the two most common symptoms are headache and depression. "Brain fog" is a classic symptom of toxic damage to the neurologic system.

(3) When the toxins damage the endocrine system, we develop obesity, diabetes, and insulin resistance.

6. Heavy metals = health problems.

We all have heavy metal toxicity. In some of us, it causes the mitochondrial damage that leads to cell apoptosis (death).[76]

Heavy metals damage the inside of our blood vessels. Heavy metals burn their way along, causing small explosions in the lining of the blood vessels as they travel through.[77] When heavy metals burn and scratch the lining of the blood vessels, the blood vessels are injured and cannot work properly anymore.[78]

This happens in all of the blood vessels from the tiniest capillaries[79] to the large blood vessels like the aorta.[80] When blood vessels are injured, many problems develop, including erectile dysfunction and impairment of mental abilities.

There is a new class of cancer-causing estrogens being called "metalloestrogens." [81] These metals have shown an ability to bind with estrogen receptors. By locking onto estrogen receptors, these metals block the good estrogen from going into the cells and doing its job to keep us healthy.

Mercury is the second most toxic element in the world.

There are no safe levels in humans. For many people, their highest toxic burden is mercury poisoning. Mercury is a common metal that is found in the food supply. Mercury toxicity may be fatal. It prevents proper brain function. Mercury accumulates, especially in the liver, brain, and kidney. There is some data linking autoimmune diseases to mercury.[82] The research is so convincing that the EPA, FDA, WHO, and United Nations Food and Agriculture Organization recommend that pregnant women, nursing mothers, and young children totally avoid all high-risk fishes and have low-risk fish no more than twice a week.

(1) The most common source of mercury is in your mouth, at least in most of us. Mercury is used in amalgam dental fillings.[83] Dental fillings with mercury are often the major cause of poor health for many people.

Currently, Sweden, Denmark, and Germany severely restrict the use of mercury amalgams. According to the EPA, mercury is a highly toxic substance that cannot legally be disposed of in a landfill. But the American Dental Association says that it is OK to put it into your mouth.

Dental research has acknowledged for many years that localized gingivitis and periodontitis (inflammation of the gums and alveolar bone loss) occur around a tooth with a "silver" amalgam, but these mercury amalgams are still put into patients' mouths by many dentists. Mercury in the amalgam vaporizes in the mouth and crosses unimpeded into the brain and across cell membranes.

A single amalgam outgasses 15 micrograms a day, more with increased chewing, and hot liquids. Daily absorption from seafood is closer to 2.3 micrograms a day. If you have mercury fillings, anytime you chew or when you drink hot liquids, you are outgassing mercury into your body where it accumulates.

(2) Mercury is concentrated in the fish we eat. In California, all of the old mines are leaching great amounts of mercury into the water table, streams, and rivers. There are high mercury emissions wherever utility plants produce electricity from fossil fuels. The cement industry releases vast amounts of mercury into the air, water, and land.

Inorganic and elemental mercury is picked up out of the water by plankton and bacteria and converted to methylmercury. This mercury is then picked up by small fish as they consume the organisms.

The small fish are then eaten by larger fish. By the time it gets into the largest fish (tuna, swordfish, shark, walleye, largemouth bass, king mackerel, northern pike) and is eaten by man, the mercury has been concentrated *over a million times* from the concentration of mercury in the water. The bigger fish, like swordfish, shark and tuna, have the most mercury. Salmon has an intermediate amount of mercury. Little sardines have the lowest amount of mercury. According to the U.S. EPA, a 25-kg child may only consume a meal of chunk white tuna once every 18.6 days to stay within safety levels for human consumption.[84]

(3) Mercury is present in some of the flu vaccines that are injected (not the nasal vaccines).[85] Injectable vaccines that contain mercury (thimerosal) may harm your immune system. When your immune system malfunctions, you fall prey to many diseases, including serious autoimmune diseases like lupus and multiple sclerosis, as well as allergies.

Lead is associated with bad behavior.[86]

Lead toxicity is one of the largest environmental medical problems in terms of numbers of people exposed and the public health toll. People in prisons have much higher levels of heavy metals than others.[87] The main target for lead toxicity is the nervous system. It is particularly destructive to children whose nervous systems are immature. Lead toxicity causes *permanent* learning and behavioral disorders. Children living in older homes who might be exposed to old lead paint or lead in the plumbing are most at risk.

Extensive research has been done documenting the toxic effects of lead on a child's learning, behavior, and social development. Lead harms the kidneys and both male and female reproduction.

Lead causes mitochondrial dysfunction. The higher the lead level, the worse the mitochondrial functioning is all over the body. The damage is even worse if alcohol is being used.[88 89] Drinking alcohol compounds your toxic burden and makes it much more difficult to remove the toxins.

Lead is still pervasive, even though it is no longer commonly used in gasoline or paint. The damage has been done. Lead persists in the soil, especially in old urban areas. When it gets hot, the lead in the soil is vaporized into the air. Our food grows in that soil. Our children play on that soil. Inner city children have the highest levels of lead because they play on soil that is highly contaminated with lead.[90]

Lead is still used in oil-based paints. It is still used in the solder in plumbing. The first water coming out of the pipes will have the most lead in it. Some hair dyes contain lead. Alcohol consumption and smoking (possibly because of contamination of tobacco leaves with lead-containing pesticides) increase the risk of elevated lead.

Cadmium is associated with breast and prostate cancer.

Tobacco smoking is the most important source of cadmium. Cigarette smokers have four to five times the cadmium level of nonsmokers and two to three times as much in the kidneys. Sources of cadmium in food are sunflower seeds, shellfish, and shrimp. Cadmium is found in many farm fertilizers, steel-belted tires, herbicides, and batteries.

Cadmium is a xenoestrogen that has been associated with higher rates of breast cancer[91] and prostate cancer.[92] Cadmium especially damages brain tissue and leads to kidney disease and cancer.[93] Cadmium is identified as a risk factor for early hardening of the arteries and hypertension. The combination of cadmium and lead is particularly damaging to the inside of the blood vessels.[94] Zinc supplements help to prevent this damage.[95]

Aluminum is high in the brains of people with Alzheimer's.[97] [98] The level of aluminum in a city's water supply directly correlates with the levels of Alzheimer's in that city. Aluminum is in lipstick, along with many other dangerous metals and chemicals.[99] If you cook with aluminum pots, the aluminum leeches right into your food and then into you. Aluminum is found in high concentrations in most tap water, because municipalities use an aluminum pan to filter out particulate matter in the final step of water purification.

Women who use antiperspirants and deodorants that contain aluminum have a much higher risk of getting breast cancer.[100] Those breast cancers often occur in the areas of the breast that rub up against the armpits, where the harmful chemicals have been applied. Use of antiperspirants and deodorants has also been linked with increased prostate cancer in men.[101]

Arsenic permeates the groundwater in the United States. Levels of arsenic in the groundwater are so high that many cities and towns cannot comply with the federal standards for arsenic.

Arsenic is in most chicken.[102] Arsenic has been deliberately added to the chicken feed because it destroys their mitochondrial function so that they don't burn fat. These fattened chickens earn more money for the chicken producers. Arsenic is in herbicides, pesticides, rice, and seafood and is used as a preservative in most wood. You will see warnings on wood used to build decks.

Arsenic has been classified as a class one carcinogen.[103] Lung cancer,[104] skin cancer,[105] bladder cancer,[106] liver cancer,[107] kidney cancer,[108] and prostate cancer[109] have all been associated with arsenic.[110] [111]

Copper, even though it is an essential trace mineral, is one of the more toxic metals. You get it from using copper utensils, copper pipes, and it is very high in drinking water. Most municipalities add copper sulfate to the drinking water to kill the algae.

7. Chemicals make us sick.

Now that we have discussed the most common heavy metals, let's examine the most common chemicals to which we are all exposed and see how they are making us sick. The fat-soluble toxic chemicals in all of our bodies are called persistent organic pollutants (POPs). Animal feeds are the main source of POPs.[112] POPs show a similarity to thyroid hormone[113] [114] and broadly act as xenotoxins.[115] [116] [117] POPs have been shown to interfere with weight loss.[118] [119]

Chlorine isn't the only bad chemical in our water. The water of every municipality in the United States contains toxic chemicals, pharmaceuticals, and heavy metals. If you want to be really shocked, ask your city or county water supplier for a printout of the chemicals found in the drinking water.

Chlorine reacts with organic materials in the water, creating chemicals that harm our health. Trihalomethanes (THMs) are toxic chemicals that result when chlorine reacts with the organic materials present in all natural waters. If you are drinking chlorinated water, you're getting THMs. Chloroform is the most well-known THM. People who ingest amounts that are high, but still below federal standards, are more likely to get cancer and have reproductive problems.[120] Trichloroacetic acid is a by-product of the chlorination of municipal water. Every city in the U.S. has a problem with this chemical. Trichloroacetic acid is associated with cancer, G.I. and liver problems, respiratory toxicity, and skin sensitivity. Those chemical facial peels are made of trichloroacetic acid.[121]

Fluoride is a neurotoxin [122] [123] that is added to most water supplies. Fluoride does not make the water safer.

Prescription drugs have found their way into our drinking water.[124] Drinking water often contains lithium, antidepressants, hormones, and a huge array of prescription drugs. The highest concentration of drugs is found downstream from water treatment plants. Water treatment plants cannot remove these pharmaceutical drugs from the water.

Pesticides poison nerves and bones.

Pesticides (used to kill bugs) were developed during World War II. At that time, scientists were put to the task of creating biochemical weapons that could be used to exterminate people. The Geneva Convention prevented the use of these toxins during war, but did not stop their development.[125] The organophosphate pesticides and pyrethrates are the two pesticide classes in most common use.

Golf courses are some of the most pesticide-contaminated places.[126] The organophosphates used on golf courses, crops, and lawns are toxic to the nerves[127] and cause abnormal bone metabolism.[128] Organophosphate toxicity can cause severe symptoms of diarrhea, excessive salivation, abnormal aggressive behavior, urinary incontinence, vomiting, muscle tremors, paralysis, and death. Organophosphates are also associated with Parkinson's disease[129] and autism.[130] The closer a person lives to fields where organophosphates are used, the more likely the person is to have autism,[131] impaired immunity, memory impairment, depression, and suicide. The Gulf War syndrome was a problem for the British and American troops who were using flea collars consisting of organophosphates.[132] [133]

We still are absorbing DDT (dichlorodiphenyltrichloroethane) *into our bodies.* DDT is a pesticide that has been proven to be so toxic that it is banned for use in the U.S. But companies are still allowed to manufacture this poison. It is exported to other countries, where it is sprayed on foods. Those DDT-laden foods are then imported back into the U.S. Eating foods sprayed with DDT is where we get most of our exposure. Whatever DDT goes into our bodies accumulates and never comes out without detoxification. DDT is so highly fat-soluble and so toxic that it is immediately bound up in the matrix and dissolved in fat stores.

Phthalates lead to infertility and cancer.

We get phthalates from eating food that contacts plastic. Wide ranges of virtually everything in our modern society have phthalates in them. Even eating food prepared by people wearing plastic gloves adds significant amounts of phthalates to the food. Phthalates are easy to ingest. The coatings on time released medications are loaded with phthalates.

Phthalates cause xenotoxicity that prevents the cells from receiving the hormones that they need to stay healthy. Xenotoxins are toxins that mimic the natural hormones that our body produces. Xenotoxins prevent us from properly metabolizing hormones.[134] These xenotoxins may just sit there blocking the doors on the cells so that the natural hormones can't come in and do their job.[135] They may stimulate the receptor in an abnormal way,[136] and their metabolites may be even more destructive. Phthalates are powerful xenoestrogens. Phthalates may cause abnormal sexual development in boys, may cause early puberty in girls and late puberty in boys, and may reduce sexual function in men. Phthalates may lead to infertility.[137] Phthalates have been associated with cancer, auto-immunity, and organ damage. Waist circumference is directly related to the amount of phthalates in the body.

Three things increase phthalates in food:
- *The longer the time phthalates are in contact with the food.*
- *The higher the fat content of the food item.*
- *Heating.*

Polyvinyl chloride may cause liver cancer.

The bottoms of plastic containers have a recycling number. If it has the number "03" on the bottom, it has phthalates and PVC. Some of the vinyl chloride will leach out of these containers into the food.[138] When it gets into your body it can cause liver cancer.[139] When these chlorine-containing containers are burned, they form dioxin, one of the most deadly chemicals ever produced.[140] PVC is commonly found in water and juice bottles and the PVC pipes that bring water into our homes. Microwaving adds phthalates and PVC to your food.

BPA is an endocrine disruptor.

BPA (Bisphenol A) is another dangerous chemical that is found in plastic. It is used extensively to manufacture commonly-used plastics and epoxy resin liners for food and beverage cans. Polycarbonate does not have phthalates, but it does contain BPA.

BPA has properties similar to diethylstilbestrol (DES). BPA has been shown to exert endocrine-disrupting effects and result in behavioral changes, altered growth, and early secondary sexual maturation. BPA is an estrogen mimicker. BPA was used as estrogen replacement for women in the 1930's, before being replaced by diethylstilbestrol.[141]

In 2010, Canada declared BPA to be a toxic substance. In Europe and Canada, BPA is no longer allowed to be used in making baby bottles. Although there is no federal program to ban BPA use in the U.S., "both the National Toxicology Program at the National Institutes of Health and FDA have some concern about the *potential effects of B.P.A. on the brain, behavior, and prostate gland in fetuses, infants, and young children.*"

The U.S. Department of Health and Human Services informs us that, "In general, plastics that are marked with recycle codes 1, 2, 4, 5, and 6 are very unlikely to contain BPA. Some, but not all, plastics that are marked with recycle codes 3 or 7 may be made with BPA."

Sunscreens damage metabolism and brain.

Sunscreens often contain ingredients that damage metabolism. We have been taught to use sunscreens to protect us from the damaging effects of the sun. But using sunscreens that contain toxic chemicals is bad for our metabolism and our health. The danger from the sunscreen may far outweigh the dangers of sun exposure.[142] Sunscreens are one example of many where an important medical treatment to prevent cancer has been perverted to become a major source of cancer. Anti-aging physicians discourage the use of skin lotions that contain chemicals that easily go into our bodies but are difficult to remove.

Nanoparticles in sunscreens and in thousands of food and health care products damage our brains. Titanium dioxide nanoparticles are commonly found in sunscreens and are also used massively in our food supply and other products. Evidence shows that they cause breaks in the DNA,[143] damage chromosomes, and increase inflammation, all of which increase the risk for cancer.[144] [145] Nanoparticles are so small that they cannot be filtered out by the cell membrane or the blood brain barrier. The blood brain barrier is designed to keep things out of our brains that could harm us. But these nanoparticles zip right into our brains, where they may be linked to Alzheimer's and Parkinson's disease.[146] They go directly into the brain and every other organ, and there is no way to keep them out or get them out. The brain is a very special organ. It cannot repair itself by replacing nerve cells. Nerve cells are particularly vulnerable to long-term, low-dose toxicity.

Oxybenzone is another carcinogenic ingredient in sunscreens. Oxybenzone is found in many sunscreens and other skin lotions. Because oxybenzone increases the body's production of free radicals and has the ability to attack our DNA, it is believed to be a contributing factor in the rise of melanoma cases in people who use sunscreen. Studies have shown that oxybenzone is a xenoestrogen that may cause breast cancer.[147] [148] Oxybenzone has also been linked to contact eczema. Oxybenzone is a dangerous chemical that was found by the CDC to be present in the urine of 96.8% of 2517 people who were tested.[149] The CDC recommends that parents avoid using anything that contains oxybenzone on their children, because of a child's inability to break it down. Oxybenzone has also been associated with low birth weight in baby girls born to women exposed to it during their pregnancies. In Europe, products with more than a half of a percent of oxybenzone in them must be labeled with "contains oxybenzone."

Oxybenzone is particularly dangerous as an ingredient in sunscreen, because serious DNA damage occurs when oxybenzone is applied to the skin and a person goes out into the sun. It has been called a "photocarcinogen" because it increases the risk of cancer when people use it and then go out in the sun.[150] It may also cause allergic dermatitis when people use it and then go out in the sun.[151] [152] [153] People complain of a burning sensation and erythema for one or a few days, and/or dermatitis with scaling lasting for up to 3 weeks.[154]

Parabens are found in breast tumors.[155]

Parabens are other deadly chemicals found in sunscreens. They also enter the body through ingestion of preservatives, the use of cosmetics, deodorants, shampoos, toothpaste, moisturizers, and processed foods like pie fillings, jams, pickles, and beer.

They are used because they are anti-fungal. Parabens have been associated with cancer.[156] Researchers found traces of parabens in tissues from twenty different kinds of breast tumors.

Hot coffee in styrofoam cups is toxic.

Styrene is another harmful contaminant found in auto exhaust, cigarette smoke, fatty foods in styrene containers, and styrofoam. If you put hot coffee, lemonade, or alcohol in a styrofoam container, the styrene will dissolve right into the liquid that you are drinking.[157] Styrene causes nausea, headache, fatigue, cancer, CNS depression, irritation of upper airways, leukopenia, and leukocytosis.

Pet shampoos make you and your pet toxic.

Pyrethrins are the active ingredient in pet shampoos. They have replaced organophosphates because they are less toxic. But they are, nevertheless, quite toxic.[158]

Pet shampoos also contain a chemical that prevents insects from breaking down the pyrethrins. It does the same thing to humans, making it impossible for the pyrethrins to be broken down in your body if you are exposed to these pet shampoos. Pyrethrins cause arrhythmias[159] and are very dangerous for the unborn offspring of pregnant women.[160]

Lice shampoos kill your cells.

Lindane leads to mitochondrial damage and apoptosis. It is harmful to the reproductive systems of both males and females.[161] Lindane is no longer allowed for use on food crops, but we may buy it in the drugstore and put it on our children's heads. It is still allowed for use in the U.S.A. to treat lice.

Dioxin in food damages all of our organs.

Dioxins are found to be present in everyone in numerous studies. Dioxins are often recognized as the most toxic class of chemicals ever invented by mankind. Dioxin is so dangerous that the EPA measures it in grams. Other toxic chemicals are measured in pounds.

Dioxins are present in Agent Orange, a defoliant used widely during the Viet Nam war. Dioxin has been used by paper companies to kill weeds after they have clear cut the forests, so that they can easily come in again and plant trees. Dioxins are still used on crops as herbicides outside the U.S. Dioxin is very difficult to remove from the environment and our bodies. Many people have died from dioxin exposure. Others have suffered widespread damage to every organ system in the body. Dioxin damages our DNA and causes birth defects in subsequent generations. Dioxin levels are high in farm-raised salmon and catfish, because they are fed food that contains dioxin. It concentrates in animals that are higher up on the food chain, like cattle. Therefore, the more beef and dairy products you consume, the more dioxin you will get.

PCBs (Polychlorinated biphenyls) are associated with childhood leukemia.[162] Part of the dioxin family, PCBs are released into waterways and onto the land. They were banned in the late 70's, after contaminating many bodies of water.

Solvents damage the mitochondria.

Solvents and alcohol damage the mitochondria, especially by reducing glutathione production.[163] Solvents and alcohol are also the chemical compounds that have been most closely associated with infertility in both males and females.[164] [165] [166] [167] Side effects from ingestion of solvents include dizziness, headaches, confusion, nausea, difficulty speaking and walking, unconsciousness, cancer, death, menstrual abnormalities, Parkinson's, Alzheimer's, autism, mitochondrial damage, and liver and kidney damage.

Tetrachloroethylene is a dry-cleaning solvent that has contaminated the groundwater in many cities. There is a phase-out program in place. But it is too late. The ground has been saturated with it. Tetrachloroethylene is found in carpet-cleaning solvents and de-greasing products. Researchers have found an association between tetrachloroethylene levels and drug-using behavior.[168] Trichloroethylene and tetrachloroethylene are found in dry-cleaning fluids, grain fumigants, de-caffeinated coffee, medications to kill hookworms, and degreasers.

Chlordane kills termites and your immunity.

Chlordane was used to treat houses for termites before 1987. So if you live in a house built before 1987, there is a good chance that you live in a chlordane-treated home. People living in a chlordane-treated home for 3-15 months have shown increased immunotoxicity and elevated levels of a number of autoantibodies including antimitochondrial antibodies (AMA).[169]

All of the North Americans who have been studied have chlordane. It is a carcinogen[170] and may cause infants born to chlordane-exposed mothers to have hormone imbalances. It is most prevalent in the soil around the foundation of a home that was treated with it.

VOCs may cause chronic fatigue.

VOCs (Volatile Organic Compounds) are liquids that evaporate into the air at normal temperatures. The toxic VOCs carry chemicals that are embedded into products to make them wrinkle-proof, stain resistant, or as glue. Often household air is imbued with many of these toxic contaminants. Formaldehyde has been shown to be toxic to many people. Common symptoms include chronic fatigue and anti-mitochondrial antibodies. NutraSweet (aspartame) is metabolized into formaldehyde.[171]

B. SICK METABOLISM FROM INFECTIOUS DISEASE.

INFECTION PREVENTS US FROM LOSING BELLY FAT. A major source of toxins is infectious disease, both the foreign agents and the many chemicals that they produce.

Americans, on the average, spend 90% of their time indoors.[172] Much of that time is spent in buildings with closed doors and closed windows. Breathing this re-circulated air exposes us to microorganisms from the skin, hair, nostrils, and mouths of other people.

We are also traveling more. Traveling exposes us to more sources of food and water that may be contaminated with pathological organisms that infect our digestive systems.

Parasites often go undetected and untreated, eventually resulting in leaky gut. Yeast is also a big problem for many people. Antibiotics result in dysbiosis and further degeneration of digestive functioning.

Many strange new viruses now infect many of us, such as Lymes coinfections, stealth viruses, Hantavirus, bird flu, swine flu, and AIDS. More common viruses such as Herpes, influenza, and upper and lower respiratory infections also present health challenges.

When your immune system can't keep viruses under control, symptoms may present continuously or periodically. Viruses underlie many diseases (like Chronic Fatigue Syndrome).

1. Bacterial infections are often present.

Infections often hide somewhere and that is predominantly in the gastrointestinal tract (GIT). Pathologic bacteria and parasites in the GIT are common and becoming more common.

Infections in the lower GIT may be a source of smoldering infection. The anus reflects the health of the GIT above. Consider hemorrhoids, anal itching, and other anal pains to be indications that the GIT is inflamed, infected, allergic, or toxic.

The most common infectious disease in developing countries is dysbiosis. Dysbiosis is the pathologic growth of "bad" bacteria in the gastrointestinal tract. The loss of normal healthy flora ("good" bacteria) in the GIT is highly destructive to your health. Drinking chlorinated tap water may create dysbiosis, although the primary cause is the use of antibiotics. Drinking tap water and eating uncooked fruits and vegetables in third-world countries may allow pathogens to enter the body. These pathogens may be able to overwhelm the defenses of the body, causing health problems which may range from mild to life-threatening. In many cases, you then carry these organisms (especially the parasites) for the rest of your life and pass them to others, unless you do a state-of-the-art GI profile to find them and then find a physician to assist you in eradicating them.

Identifying infections at the top of the GIT (your mouth) is of paramount importance. Good dental hygiene is essential for health. Treat gum infections before they become more serious with the appearance of cavities, tooth abscesses, or bone erosion. The most common source of heart valve infections is oral disease and infection.

Bacterial balance on the skin (skin flora) is important. Health depends upon keeping the good bacteria balanced with pathological bacteria. The skin is your largest organ. You need to have healthy bacteria on your skin in order to prevent disease. The use of anti-bacterial soaps, lotions, and gels not only puts potent toxins into your body, but it kills the good bacteria and creates space for a dysbiosis to occur on your skin.

Anti-aging physicians recommend against using toxic chemicals on your skin. Traditional MDs are beginning to understand the dangers of toxic chemicals and the importance of a balanced flora both on the skin and in the GIT. We must also keep in mind that the production of toxic chemicals is not good for the environment.

Infection in the sinuses causes sick metabolism. Chronic infection in the sinuses (the top of the respiratory tract) may be minimally symptomatic, but damages the metabolism with smoldering inflammation. Often structural problems are present, causing decreased vitality in the tissues of the sinuses. Structural problems in the head are often the result of birth trauma, auto accidents, and other head trauma.

Chronic irritation from pollutants or allergies predisposes to chronic infection. Decongestant drugs used to treat allergies dry the mucous throughout the entire body, which thickens secretions in the sinuses and lungs. *Infection hides in these dried secretions.* Decongestants also have side effects that affect the brain and other tissues. Decongestant drugs are toxins that the body must detoxify and remove.

2. Viral infections are increasing.

When your immune system is weak, chronic viruses may become active and cause symptoms like sore throats and fatigue. As your immune system gets weaker, the viral injury increases. The viruses go right into the DNA of your cells and replicate. It is important to eliminate viruses if you want to enjoy superior health. Otherwise you are always fighting viral infection.

Lymes disease is a combination of Borrelia infection (bacterial) and a number of co-infections that cross over the boundaries of virus, parasite, and bacteria, including Bartonella, Babesia (a red blood cell parasite), Anaplasma, and Ehrlichia.

To make things impossibly difficult, Lymes disease is strongly immunosuppressive. In chronic Lymes patients, the blood tests that initially showed the infection turn negative.

Opportunistic diseases like the fatigue viruses (EBV, HHV-6, HSV-1), Borna disease virus, mycoplasma, mold, and yeast greatly compound the disease state and toxic state of the Lyme patient and complicate the diagnostic picture.

"Stealth viruses" are responsible for many illnesses. In the same way that AIDS was unidentified when it emerged in the late 70's and early 80's, "stealth viruses" are becoming very common and causing illness like Chronic Fatigue Syndrome (CFS). They are called stealth viruses because they have not yet been identified.

Stealth viruses are implicated in some cases of Parkinson's, and are responsible for many other diseases. Stealth viruses may present very differently in many people and cause a variety of disease states.

3. Parasites are often undiagnosed.

Parasites may be the cause of recurring mild abdominal discomfort, gas, and loose stools. They are often contracted when traveling to third-world countries. Even in first-world countries, parasites get into the public food and water supply. Chlorine kills bacteria, but not parasites.

Typically, symptoms include diarrhea and abdominal pain. In some people, their immune systems can overcome the parasites, but often medication is required to eliminate them.

People often believe that they are safe from parasites if they wash their hands before preparing food, don't eat poorly cooked pork, and avoid drinking tap water and eating raw fruits and vegetables when traveling to foreign countries. But parasites are often contracted by people who scrupulously do all these things.

When you eat out, you don't know if the person who prepared your salad washed their hands before preparing it. A pork dish with a spicy sauce may hide inadequately cooked pork.

Parasitic disease saps people's vitality until they die, or until they get tested and the parasite is correctly identified and treated. Whatever the story, the result is the same. A person may get an acute stomach upset for a few days and some diarrhea. Then he feels OK and thinks that he must have had the stomach flu. A month later, he has forgotten this when he gets unexplained mild abdominal discomfort and looseness of stool. After a week of Pepto-Bismol and Imodium, he feels mostly OK. Then a month later, this reoccurs. It is mild, nothing to worry about, but it just keeps happening. This is a common presentation of parasites. The "turista" in Mexico normally is a dysbiosis from Mexican GI flora. But in some cases, it is due to amoebic dysentery, an inflammation of the intestine due to infection with the parasitic amoeba, entamoeba histolytica, or other parasites.

Anti-aging physicians are aware of diseases that disrupt the integrity of the intestinal lining, which lead to multiple food allergies and high states of inflammation. When these diseases are not treated, systemic complications may develop, like liver abscesses, brain cysts, or lung involvement.

4. Leaky gut leads to food allergies.

The most common cause for "leaky gut" is untreated parasitic disease. When our digestive tract has an intact barrier, food proteins do not leak across into the blood. But if the barrier begins to leak, we call it "leaky gut."[173] Leaky gut syndrome is caused by damage to the linings of the intestine and leads to multiple food allergies. Parasites may cause leaky gut.[174][175] Food antigens, bacterial toxins, and other infectious agents can get into the body through the leaky gut and produce inflammation.[176]

Proinflammatory cytokines then perpetuate a vicious cycle of chronic inflammation. The inflammation also happens in the brain. It becomes very difficult to get out of this vicious cycle. When the blood brain barrier becomes compromised, major depression or fatigue may result.[177] Immune system function is also severely harmed by leaky gut.[178]

5. Undiagnosed yeast infections are common.

Yeast infections are widely prevalent in our society, but few people are aware that yeast is what is causing their health problems. An overgrowth of the yeast organism, candida albicans, causes a dysbiosis, or imbalance of intestinal flora. It most commonly begins as a result of antibiotic usage.

Candida albicans puts out a very potent toxin, acetaldehyde. It can produce very serious and even life-threatening disease and can mimic a host of serious pathologies.

C. SICK METABOLISM FROM HORMONAL IMBALANCE.

*I*F YOUR HORMONES DON'T WORK, YOU GET FAT. Both men and women often gain fat, especially toxic belly fat, as they enter the change of life and hormone balance shifts. *Unless insulin, cortisol, DHEA, thyroid, estrogen, progesterone, testosterone, and growth hormone are brought into the healthy range (not what is normal for an older person), weight loss strategies will be ineffective in the long term.*

1. Toxic belly fat = insulin resistance.

Overeating of carbohydrates produces belly fat and sets off a chain of events leading to metabolic syndrome and eventually to diabetes. Snacking on carbohydrate foods provides no notice to the body of satiety, so the body is urged on to endless consumption of carbohydrates. The excessively high glycemic loads in carbohydrate snacks cause sugar to supersaturate the tissues. This sugar supersaturation produces toxic glycosylated end products (GEP). The snack food companies encourage this mindless overconsumption by adding salt, preservatives, and artificial colors and flavors which further damage our metabolism. The end result is the infamous metabolic syndrome or Syndrome X.

Metabolic syndrome may cause high blood pressure. Adiposity, toxicity, and deposition of glycosylated end products produce a total body degenerative disease process. The person with metabolic syndrome has increased belly fat (and chest fat), abnormal fats in the blood (dyslipidemia), hypertension, and insulin resistance. The sustained high glucose and insulin levels affect the number and sensitivity of insulin receptors. Increased glucose and free fatty acids (FFAs) produce increased insulin. Increased insulin increases sodium reabsorption and activation of the sympathetic nervous system (contributing to the hypertension along with the increased inflammatory chemicals).

Fat cells (adipocytes) produce substances called "adipokines" that make it hard to lose weight. As toxic belly fat accumulates, these adipokines become unbalanced. Then it becomes more difficult to lose weight, and health deteriorates.

Fat cells produce these adipokines:

1. Enzymes.

a. **Aromatase** turns testosterone to estrogen. Aromatase is responsible for the formation of the "beer belly" and flabby breast tissue of men as they gain toxic belly fat. As testosterone turns into estrogen, they are becoming feminized. Elevated estrogen levels lead to prostate inflammation and estrogen dominance.

b. **11-Beta-HSD1** (11-beta-hydroxysteroid dehydrogenase 1) contributes to the formation of metabolic syndrome.[179]

2. Hormones.[180]

a. **Leptin** is the energy-balancing hormone. In obesity, the cells become oblivious to it, and appetite becomes unregulated.

b. **Estrogen** is formed from testosterone by aromatase. In men, too much estrogen leads to prostate problems. In menopausal women, when the ovaries stop producing estrogen, more belly fat appears in order to make more estrogen to try to pick up the slack. This contributes to estrogen dominance.

c. **Adiponectin** is the good hormone. It increases insulin sensitivity. Levels are low in fat people and high in thin people. Decreased expression of adiponectin is correlated with insulin resistance.[181]

d. **Angiotensinogen** is a hormone involved in hypertension (high blood pressure).

e. **Resistin** contributes to insulin resistance.

f. **Retinol-binding protein 4** (RBP4) [182] contributes to insulin resistance.

3. Inflammatory cytokines. These are chemicals that act on other cells to produce inflammation, drive many degenerative diseases, and impair healthy metabolism.

a. **TNF-alpha** (Tumor Necrosis Factor Alpha). TNF-alpha *activates the whole inflammatory sequence.* TNF-alpha creates insulin resistance and increased free fatty acids.

b. **IL-6** (Interleukin 6) is a major inflammatory cytokine of the interleukin series.

4. Complement factors.

a. **Factor D** (adipsin) increases fat and is elevated in obesity.

b. **Prothrombic agents.** PAI-1 (Plasminogen Activating Inhibitor Factor-1) leads to deep venous thrombosis, stroke, and heart attacks. PAI-1 increases in obesity and metabolic syndrome.

5. Substrates.

a. **Free fatty acids** contribute to insulin resistance in muscle and metabolic syndrome.

b. **Glycerol** is converted to glucose in the liver.

2. Adrenal dysfunction and cortisol.

The adrenals release hormones that deal with stress. Adrenal dysfunction is primarily caused by too much mental, emotional, and physical stress. Adrenal dysfunction is defined as the overproduction of stress hormones or the inability of the adrenal glands to produce adequate amounts of stress hormones in a normal daily rhythm.

All of the other hormones of the body depend on optimal functioning of the adrenals. When the adrenals are dysfunctional, degeneration of the body organs occurs. Poor adrenal function especially impairs the brain and heart, and thyroid and sex hormones. Improving adrenal function will automatically improve thyroid and sex hormones without making any other changes.

- **Cortisol is a stress hormone produced by the adrenals.**
- **Cortisol maintains blood pressure.**
- **Cortisol maintains blood sugar.**
- **Cortisol reduces inflammation.**

A normal daily pattern is a peak of cortisol levels in the morning, decreasing throughout the day, and low at night. When the adrenals are functioning well, there is a spike of cortisol at 8 AM. This is the stimulus for the body to wake up and get going for the day's activities. In a healthy cycle, as cortisol levels drop to near zero at midnight, this gives the signal for the hormonal sequencing of sleep, internal cleansing, and regeneration, especially the brain.

When the adrenals become dysfunctional, this pattern changes. Stress initially causes high cortisol at all hours of the day (especially at night). When cortisol is high all the time, it encourages insulin resistance and weight gain, especially in the abdominal area. This toxic belly fat contributes to chronic inflammation, increasing the risk for heart disease. This toxic belly fat also produces excess estrogen. Increased estrogen decreases thyroid function, causing further weight gain.

Continuously high cortisol burns up the building blocks of the body and creates abdominal fat by stimulating the appetite.

(1) The immune system becomes depressed.

(2) High cortisol increases appetite. When sustained stress keeps cortisol levels high, the cortisol will cause the body to refuel when it doesn't need to refuel. *This excess cortisol production stimulates glucose production, because cortisol is an important mechanism for elevating blood sugar when you get hypoglycemic.* Cortisol produced during fight or flight reactions will first burn carbohydrates for quick energy. When the immediate stress is over, the cortisol increases the appetite to replace those carbohydrates that it just burned. If the person uses stimulants and does *not* eat, this is the fastest way to burn out the adrenals.

(3) Excess cortisol produces deficient serotonin, resulting in sugar cravings.[183] [184]

(4) Cortisol is catabolic. This means that it breaks down tissues. When it is high all the time, it causes a breakdown in the muscles, bones, connective tissue, and brain.

As the adrenal dysfunction progresses, the adrenals become exhausted and cortisol levels will drop at all hours of the day. *As the adrenals become burned out, (stage 4 dysfunction) they can barely produce enough cortisol to support the normal activities of life.* If you have chronic stress, a major illness, or trauma, DHEA will be stolen from its job in making sex hormones and will be used to make cortisol. Without enough sex hormones, you won't have much sexual interest or function.

Mild and moderate dysfunction (Stage 1-4) is not recognized by traditional medicine. Only Addison's disease (total non-function of the adrenals) and Cushing's disease (extreme hyperfunction) are recognized by most physicians.

But the stages of mild and moderate dysfunction are extremely important to understand and treat in order to improve the health of many sick people. When stress is prolonged, it may lead to adrenal fatigue and eventually to adrenal exhaustion, neither of which are recognized by traditional doctors as treatable medical conditions.

Stage 1 adrenal stress is when cortisol and adrenalin are high. In stage one adrenal dysfunction, the stress hormones become elevated all the time. People in stage 1 have elevated blood sugar levels, because they're pumping out lots of cortisol. Doctors would call it a diabetic profile of glucose utilization. This means that the person is becoming insulin-resistant. Insulin resistance causes more fat to be distributed onto the abdomen.

They have insomnia. They are anxious. They are hyper. A lot of young people are in this stage for years. They work long hours but they're still going strong. They don't complain of fatigue. They are addicted to adrenalin and stimulants. If they continue on with this high-stress life, they will move on to Stage 2, 3, and 4.

Stage 2-3 adrenal fatigue is where the cortisol reserves are dropping. Cortisol levels are low and adrenals can't keep up anymore. People with adrenal fatigue wake up tired in the morning. One difference between adrenal fatigue and thyroid fatigue is that thyroid fatigue usually makes people tired in afternoon. With adrenal fatigue people are tired the entire day, until the evening.

Stage 3-4 adrenal exhaustion is when reserves are low or completely depleted. In adrenal exhaustion your body is exhausting its cortisol. Cortisol is very low and all the precursor hormones are low. Energy drops and it becomes difficult to perform normal activities. There is a need for immediate treatment.

3. DHEA is anabolic and balances cortisol.

- **DHEA helps to repair damaged cells.**
- **DHEA boosts the immune system.**
- **DHEA levels should be monitored.**
- **DHEA is a precursor of sex hormones.**
- **DHEA can be prescribed in cream from compounded pharmacies for best absorption.**

- **The most common side effect of too much DHEA is excessive androgens, which may cause acne or masculinizing side effects, like facial hair in women.**

Women who are low in DHEA stop shaving their legs because there is no hair there anymore. Men who are low in DHEA notice that the leg hair completely stops below the sock line. They may think that the socks have rubbed the hair off.

DHEA targets fat loss around the abdomen. DHEA causes weight loss by raising the metabolic thermostat, causing you to burn more energy. If you are low in DHEA you will feel colder. It stimulates enzymes in the liver responsible for thermogenesis (burning calories). DHEA is higher in thinner people and lower in fatter people.

When DHEA is optimized, it promotes a sense of well-being. As it is depleted, serotonin metabolism is affected. As serotonin levels drop, carbohydrate cravings increase, leading to more weight gain.

The loss of DHEA decreases sex drive. DHEA peaks in the early twenties, dropping steeply after age 40, more so in people under stress, and declining to very low levels by the age of seventy. When DHEA drops, it accentuates the loss of the sex hormones. It is important to keep levels up, because the sex hormones are formed from it.

DHEA prevents wrinkles by building collagen. By having sufficient reserves of DHEA, you decrease wrinkles. To test your collagen, pinch the back of your hand to see how fast your skin springs back.

DHEA repairs damaged memory. The neuron connections (dendrites) help with associative thinking. Aging and excessive cortisol cause dendrites to retract, but DHEA can repair them.[185] DHEA also acts as an antidepressant.

DHEA keeps people sexually attractive, improves quality of life, and reduces mortality from all causes.[186] It improves cognition and protects the immune system. DHEA is anabolic—it builds tissue. It stimulates the immune system, and maintains tissue elasticity and repair. DHEA lowers heart disease[187] and protects against midlife changes. It is used in the treatment of aging, menopause, andropause, immune deficiencies, breast cancer, AIDS, and osteoporosis.

Make sure that you are taking enough sulfur. 95% of the body's DHEA is bound to sulfur molecules in the form of DHEA-S (DHEA Sulfate). MSM will do the trick. The body takes DHEA from the storage depot of DHEA-S as it needs it.

4. Improve thyroid function.

Long-term thyroid dysfunction may make you fat,[188] *and impairs and shortens your life.* By lowering your metabolism, hypothyroidism ages you faster and weakens your immune system, making you prone to infectious disease, cancer, adrenal fatigue, low stomach acid, auto-immune disorders, and cognitive (memory) problems. When thyroid levels are low, people often gain weight and feel fatigued, especially in the afternoon. Decreased thyroid is also responsible for dry skin, thinning hair, decreased muscle mass, and aging.

Adrenal dysfunction decreases the body's ability to utilize thyroid hormone. Adrenal issues must be treated first, before the thyroid. If you treat the thyroid without treating the adrenals, you may feel worse than ever, because you are stressing an already over-stressed system that can't respond to stress properly. Often, correcting adrenal dysfunction will correct a sluggish thyroid.

In the final stages of adrenal dysfunction, *when cortisol levels drop* due to adrenal exhaustion, there is not enough cortisol to allow the thyroid hormones to do their job of increasing energy and keeping metabolism up. *Adrenal deficiency causes fatigue, low blood sugar, weight loss, and menstrual dysfunction.*

Toxicity may compromise your thyroid function. The enzymes that convert the storage form of thyroid hormone, T4, to the active form of thyroid hormone, T3, are negatively affected by *drugs, toxins, dieting, stress, trauma, and zinc or selenium deficiency.* Toxicity may block the formation of T3, which is used to make energy in every cell in the body.

In an estrogen-dominant state, thyroid hormone function is diminished because estrogen increases thyroid-binding globulin, which binds free thyroid hormone. *This creates fatigue and weight gain.* Thyroid function may normalize when natural bioidentical progesterone (available only by prescription) is used to treat the estrogen dominance.

5. Leptin and ghrelin backfire.

The hormone "leptin" is produced by belly fat and "ghrelin" is produced by the stomach. Let's see how leptin and ghrelin control our appetite and energy use. Then we will see how the balance of leptin and ghrelin is disturbed by excess belly fat. With excess belly fat, leptin and ghrelin go haywire, causing us to be unable to lose the belly fat.

The brain has two centers that control hunger:
- ## The feeding center.
- ## The satiety center.

The hypothalamus in the brain has a feeding center that is always active and a satiety center that acts to inhibit the feeding center. Leptin and ghrelin rule these centers.

Leptin

Leptin (meaning thin in Greek) activates the satiety center and inhibits the feeding center. Fat is the primary producer of leptin. Leptin tells your brain that you don't need to eat any more and also that you need to get moving. When you stop eating and start exercising, the fat is used for energy. When the fat is used, leptin drops, and you feel hungry.

It's a great feedback system when it works. But too much belly fat damages the leptin system. In obese individuals, leptin stops working the way it should. The leptin is there, but it doesn't work anymore. In obese individuals, the belly fat produces *very high leptin levels.*

High, sustained concentrations of leptin close the leptin doors (receptors) on the cells in the brain. Leptin can't come in anymore.[189] This is called leptin resistance.

Now the brain center for satiety doesn't work anymore, and the feeding center stays on. When leptin doesn't work anymore, you stay hungry, you never get satisfied, you eat more and more, and you get fatter and fatter.

Ghrelin and adiponectin.

Ghrelin is the opposing factor to leptin and increases hunger by stimulating the feeding center and inhibiting the satiety center. Ghrelin is a hormone primarily released by the stomach that increases hunger.

It has been used with anorexics to get them to eat.[190] It is speculated that excess belly fat may increase sensitivity to ghrelin. When there is too much belly fat, there may be more ghrelin receptors (doors) that allow ghrelin to come into the brain cells to stimulate the feeding center and inhibit the satiety center, so not as much ghrelin is needed to stimulate hunger.[191]

Adiponectin is another hormone produced by belly fat, but it is inappropriately low in obesity. It produces insulin sensitivity, lipid oxidation, and has important vascular protection effects and anti-inflammatory actions. PCB toxicity may be one cause for low adiponectin levels.[192]

6. Progesterone in females.

Adequate progesterone levels are crucial to a woman's health. Progesterone reduces insulin levels and helps to regulate blood sugar levels. Progesterone is beneficial to the cardiovascular system and to balance the effects of estradiol. Progesterone builds strong bones. Progesterone is neuroprotective. We have progesterone receptors in the brain, breast, bone, heart and many other organs. In the breast, progesterone up-regulates estrogen receptors. In the brain, progesterone increases GABA, the calming neurotransmitter. Progesterone has been used to treat traumatic brain injury, acne, as a contraceptive, in menopause, for PMS, for some menstrual disorders, to inhibit prostate growth, and for problems with pregnancy.

Stress drops progesterone levels. Progesterone drops in women even before they reach menopause. If a woman is under constant stress, her adrenals are always pumping out cortisol. Cortisol is made from 17-hydroxyprogesterone. High levels of stress hormones may lead to a progesterone-deficient state where estrogen dominates. When progesterone is deficient, unopposed estrogen may build to unsafe tissue levels that may lead to breast cancer and other reproductive organ cancers.

7. Estrogen in females.

Estrogen deficiency.

The health of every cell, tissue, organ, and organ system in the female depends on an adequate supply of estrogen. Estradiol or E2 has about four hundred functions that are important to maintaining good health.

When women enter menopause, their estrogen levels drop and they become estrogen-deficient. In menopause, the ovaries stop producing estradiol. Loss of estradiol in menopause causes many metabolic changes. When estrogen drops in menopause, women develop the symptoms of hormone deficiency--deterioration in the health of the body, including brain function, heart function, and bone density.

Thinner women usually have less estrogen. Chronic dieters, anorexics, and overtrained women athletes often have low estrogen levels. A woman may be estrogen-deficient (low estrogen) and estrogen-dominant (too much estrogen when compared to progesterone) at the same time.

Estrogen dominance.

Estrogen dominance occurs when the sum of all the body's estrogens is too high in relation to progesterone. The body's estrogens include E1 (estrone), E2 (estradiol), E3 (estriol), *plus* estrogen metabolites, xenoestrogens, dietary estrogens, and any estrogens from hormone replacement therapy (HRT) and birth control estrogens. The most common pre-menopausal hormone imbalance is estrogen excess and progesterone deficiency.

The estrogen-dominant woman is irritable and bloated. Without progesterone, estrogen allows water and sodium to come into the cells. At the same time, potassium and magnesium are lost from the cells, and the electrolyte balance is upset. Too much copper is retained and too much zinc is lost.[193]

Estrogen excess prevents weight loss by decreasing metabolism. In an estrogen-excess state, thyroid hormone function is diminished because estrogen increases thyroid-binding globulin, which binds free thyroid hormone. *This creates fatigue and weight gain.* Allergies may worsen. Blood clots more easily which may set you up for a stroke or embolism. Bile thickens and gallbladder problems develop.

Estrogen dominance is often exacerbated by lack of exercise, poor diet and lifestyle choices, use of birth control pills, Premarin, and toxicity caused by environmental toxins that are being taken in and stored in the body. Add to this the decreased ability of the body to metabolize and excrete the estrogen it produces. Obesity contributes to estrogen dominance, because the fat cells produce estrogen. As the years go by, the estrogen-dominant state and its symptoms worsen.

8. Testosterone in females.

Testosterone may be too high. It is important to have a correct ratio between estrogen and testosterone levels. In menopause, the ovaries stop producing estrogen, but continue to produce the androgen, androstenedione. She may develop symptoms of high androgens (including testosterone) in proportion to estrogen, becoming more masculinized, growing facial hair, pushy behavior, and getting more acne.

Testosterone may be too low. If the ovaries are removed, androgen levels drop to half. Low androgen levels may occur at other times, too. Low androgen levels lead to low libido, depression, memory loss, bone loss, and incontinence. Low testosterone in women may be associated with failure of the ovary, pituitary deficiency, or adrenal steal (low DHEA).

9. Testosterone in males.

When a man enters andropause, the drop in his hormones is not usually as sudden as that of a woman entering menopause, but the effects are just as devastating. Men don't have as much energy, can't think as well, muscles are weaker, and joints ache. They are depressed, moody, and lose sexual desire and function. Memory and intelligence decrease. Dementia and Alzheimer's increase. Visible changes appear as wrinkles, loss of muscle mass, and loss of height due to loss of bone density and weakened connective tissue.

Testosterone levels begin dropping after age 30 and drop off drastically in men after age 60. Half of healthy men between the ages of 50-70 will have a bioavailable testosterone level below the lowest level seen in healthy men who are 20-40.[194] A healthy 60-year-old would be a sick 25-year-old.

To add to the problem, average (regardless of age) testosterone levels are declining world-wide. Perhaps it is being caused by environmental pollution and xenoestrogens.

10. Estrogen in males.

Too much estrogen may be a problem for men. As testosterone drops, much of what is left is changed into estrogen, especially with toxic belly fat. Enzymes (aromatases) in this toxic belly fat turn their testosterone into estrogen. Although men need some estrogen, too much estrogen is not good. It opposes what little testosterone they do have.

Estrogen-dominant men may develop breast enlargement (gynecomastia) and experience prostate inflammation and swelling. As men take in xenoestrogens, produce estrogen from body fat, produce the ugly 16-hydroxy estrogen metabolites, and lose testosterone with aging, they become estrogen-dominant (in relation to testosterone).

The hormones in the toxic belly fat perpetuate a vicious cycle making men fatter and more feminine. This shift towards more estrogen and less testosterone may cause him to become less dominant and more receptive in his relationship.

11. HGH declines with age.

Human Growth Hormone (HGH) builds muscle mass, increases bone density, and burns body fat. HGH declines with age. At 60 years of age, the individual may have 25% of the HGH he had at age 20. After age 20, call HGH "repair" hormone. The decline of HGH with age is directly related to many of the symptoms of aging. HGH deficiency contributes to earlier death.

Human Growth Hormone interacts with every other hormone. HGH makes all the other hormones work by upregulating the receptors. It increases the number of receptors on the cells for estrogen, progesterone, pregnenolone, and every other hormone. HGH increases estrogen and testosterone. Need for replacement of other hormones may be eliminated or reduced when replacing growth hormone.

12. Estrogen metabolism & cancer.

When we can't properly metabolize estrogen, we become more susceptible to diseases, especially cancer.[195] Poor estrogen metabolism is associated with higher body fat and lower lean muscle.[196] This is true for both men and women. Both sexes may fall prey to cancers of the reproductive organs when estrogen metabolism is poor.[197][198]

Hydroxylation of estrogens occurs in Phase I detoxification. Xenoestrogens and horse estrogens (Premarin) are detoxified in Phase I of liver detoxification. When there is a lot of exposure to these toxins, the liver may become overwhelmed. In Phase I, if the liver is incapable of metabolizing estrogen via the good pathway (2-OH), estrogen will go down the bad (4-OH) and ugly (16-OH) pathways.[199] When estrogen is metabolized down the bad and ugly pathways, cancer becomes more likely.[200]

Estrogens are methylated in Phase II. The estrogen metabolites cannot be excreted from the body until they are methylated. In methylation, a methyl group is added to the molecule. For this to happen, you have to have a methyl group to add on, and you have to have the enzymes that will do the work. If your estrogen metabolism test shows that you are a poor methylator, you have impaired methylation throughout your metabolic pathways.

13. Neurotransmitter imbalances.

Neurotransmitters are substances that transmit signals from one nerve ending to the next. The brain communicates with the rest of the body by sending impulses between the nerves using neurotransmitters to tell us to feel good or bad, happy or sad.

When neurotransmitter levels become balanced, antidepressants or other mood-affecting pharmaceuticals may become unnecessary. Chronic inflammation and immune disorders may lead to a wide variety of clinical complaints such as depression, anxiety, insomnia, fatigue, and attention issues. Imbalances in the immune system may affect neurotransmitter levels, which may be a contributing factor to psychological complaints.

Serotonin, the master neurotransmitter, affects our mood. *Balance serotonin levels in order to balance the other neurotransmitters.* Serotonin regulates the release of dopamine, norepinephrine and glutamate. Women have more serotonin than men, and serotonin affects them more. Serotonin may lower anxiety. Serotonin may encourage closeness.

Normalizing serotonin levels is the first step in normalizing weight and feeling great. Normal serotonin levels lead to contentment, well-being, focused concentration, and ability to sleep well. Repeated dieting, stimulants, and drugs cause unbalanced serotonin levels which may lead to the inability to concentrate, depression, and sleep difficulties. Low serotonin levels cause cravings for sweets and carbohydrates, which will raise serotonin rapidly. *Often, after following a low-carb or no-carb diet for a while, low serotonin causes* craving for sweets, and the urge to eat carbohydrates will rule over the best laid plans. This leads to carbohydrate binging.

When estrogen levels drop with menopause, serotonin receptors in the brain are impaired and reduce the ability of serotonin to come into the cells.[201][202] Low serotonin levels may further lower estrogen and testosterone.

Acetylcholine gives short-term memory and muscle contractions. Without enough acetylcholine, you lose your memory. Typical decrease begins at age 40.

Dopamine motivates you to seek pleasure. *It increases sex drive and orgasms.* All drugs of addiction, like cocaine, cigarettes, and alcohol, raise and then deplete dopamine. Dopamine decreases the craving for these addictive substances. Schizophrenics often have too much. It may be used to treat Parkinson's disease, addictions, sex drive disorders, and aging. Dopamine levels begin to drop at age 30. When estrogen drops, dopamine drops.

GABA (gamma-aminobutyric acid) lowers brain excitability. GABA calms you and puts you to sleep. GABA decreases begin around age 50. Progesterone is highly effective in elevating GABA levels. When GABA drops, brain cells become more excitable.

Step II. GET STATE-OF-THE-ART TESTING.

STATE-OF-THE-ART MEDICAL TESTING *is usually done by specialty laboratories and is not available in community or hospital laboratories.* State-of-the-art medical testing uses sophisticated testing methods that are not currently available in community labs.

State-of-the-art medical testing is important in order to:
(1) Exclude serious illness.
(2) Direct your physician to make a correct diagnosis and render effective treatment.
(3) Identify current toxic exposure, so that you can stop the exposure and recover health.

In order to assess what is causing sick metabolism, it is necessary to pinpoint problems using specialized tests. Many of the diseases that cause sick metabolism have systemic complications, like the parasite complications of liver abscesses, brain cysts, or lung involvement. It is important to do the right tests in order to properly diagnose and treat disease *before* it becomes serious. The specialty laboratories providing state-of-the-art medical testing are few in number, but they are outstanding in their methodology, accuracy, and reputation.

Certainly, there are many important tests that can be done accurately by mainstream laboratories. But often doctors do *only* these tests and find nothing wrong. The problem is that the patient still does not feel well. In these cases, we need to consider more carefully what is happening on a nutritional and biochemical basis to understand what is affecting the patient's health and functioning. State-of-the-art testing using specialty labs gives us the information that we need to uncover the exact causes of health problems.

Don't expect your traditional doctor to understand or recognize the importance of all of the testing which we recommend in this book. Medical care in the U.S. revolves around the "standard of care" that is dictated by what insurance companies and managed care will pay for. Because state-of-the-art medical testing is not standard of care, most physicians have never even heard of these tests or their importance in maintaining optimal health.

Even if a patient would benefit from state-of-the-art medical testing, insurance companies and managed care usually won't pay for these tests, therefore most physicians are reluctant or unable to order them. (But the tide *is* turning and occasional testing *is* covered by insurance companies, even Medicare.)

The goal of anti-aging medicine is to exclude disease or find the disease when it is mild to moderate and not wait until the disease is extreme and causing a lot of damage. Anti-aging physicians realize that picking up disease and hormonal imbalances that are mild or moderate is what we must do if we want to age well and increase not only longevity but also quality of life. Part of this approach is to screen for and exclude diseases like intestinal parasites, where we are paying for evaluations that we hope are negative (normal).

Get the testing that you need, not just to survive, but to thrive. No one can go wrong to order testing when it is correctly done by a state-of-the-art medical testing laboratory. The testing is non-invasive and risk-free. Negative testing can reassure you that a disease state is not present. Positive testing can lead you to find a knowledgeable physician who can make a correct diagnosis. You can only go wrong by not getting the testing. If you don't take care of the problem now, your health may deteriorate, and your medical bills may mount.

Your test results will help to guide you to the right physician who is able to interpret the results, diagnose disease and its complications, and treat effectively. Your physician will now be in a much better position to help you, since many problems have been excluded and others identified. State-of-the-art testing for sick metabolism requires a physician who is knowledgeable in interpreting the results, who can make an accurate diagnosis, and who can effectively treat diseases, whether they are mild, moderate, or severe. Effective treatment for infectious disease, toxicity, and hormone imbalances depends on accurate assessment.

If you are unable to find a physician in your area who is willing to order the tests that you need, DrHormone.org can assist you to find out where you can get the necessary testing and to find a physician who can accurately diagnose and effectively treat YOUR causes of sick metabolism.

Minimal comprehensive evaluation:

This is the basic testing protocol. We will go into more detail about testing for the causes of sick metabolism in the sections that follow.

(1) Start with the gut. Health begins in the gut. Stool samples should be evaluated in a specialty lab for evidence of infection and poor digestion.

(2) Screen with testing for oxidative stress damage – Start with lipid peroxidase and DNA-repair product, 8-hydroxydeoxyguanosine (8-OHdG).

(3) If oxidative damage testing is positive, look for heavy metals and chemical toxins.

Check for heavy metals. If you have a history of exposure to heavy metals or positive testing for oxidative stress damage:

(a) Get a hair analysis and urine for heavy metals OR

(b) Get a chelated urine test from a specialty lab. You must see a physician to get the chelating agent – DMSA, DMPS, or EDTA.

Check for chemical toxicity. If you have an exposure history or positive oxidative stress damage, get the organic acid test from a specialty lab to find out where the metabolism is blocked. You may also test for specific chemical toxins.

(4) Evaluate adrenals, hypothalamus, pituitary, and growth hormone.
- Always check the adrenals first. Cortisol levels in the saliva at 8 am, noon, 5 pm, and 11pm and a DHEAS will reveal the diurnal cortisol pattern and the stage of adrenal dysfunction.
- Screen hypothalamus and pituitary function with an 8 am serum cortisol and ACTH.
- The ACTH stimulation test measures the adrenal response to adrenocorticotropic hormone (ACTH). ACTH is a hormone produced in the pituitary gland that stimulates the adrenal glands to release cortisol. This test is only done in the doctor's office.
- Test growth hormone level with a serum IGF-1 test.

(5) Next check the thyroid gland (available in community labs):
- Serum TSH.
- Total and Free T4.
- Total and Free T3, Reverse T3.
- TPO and TBG antibodies.
- Take body temperature several times during the day for a week (starting three hours after you get up). Use a glass thermometer for accuracy and write down your results.

(6) In women, check sex hormones (available in community labs): In women in their active, reproductive years, and those on cyclic BHRT, measure peak estradiol on day 12 and peak progesterone on day 21. For those on creams, use saliva to measure estrogen and progesterone.
- Serum FSH.
- Serum LH.
- Serum estradiol.

- Serum progesterone.
- Serum testosterone.
- Serum DHEA-S.

(7) To check sex hormone levels in men (available in community labs) draw:
- A serum total and free testosterone.
- Serum total estrogen.
- Serum LH.
- Serum DHEA-S.
- In men with erectile dysfunction and in all older males, add PSA and prolactin.

(8) General testing in both sexes (available in community labs) includes:
- Fasting blood sugar and fasting insulin.
- Advanced lipid profile.
- Homocysteine.
- High sensitivity CRP.
- Estrogen metabolism testing is necessary on *all* men and women (available only from state-of-the-art medical testing labs).

A. TEST FOR TOXICITY.

*E*VERYONE SHOULD GET SCREENED FOR HEAVY METALS AND CHEMICAL TOXICITY. Oxidative stress testing and mitochondrial damage assessment are screening tools for assessing damage from heavy metals and chemical toxicity. Porphyrin testing screens for ongoing damage and sick metabolism from a specific list of toxins. If you have an exposure history, test for that specific toxin.

1. Test oxidative damage and screen for toxicity.

The oxidative damage assessment test and organic acid tests available from specialty labs are good screening tests for most chronic illnesses. Toxic metals and chemicals usually create oxidative damage as part of their toxic effects on the human body. These are good tests to use to find the extent of toxic damage. When used as an adjunct to the clinical history, test results may be used to guide the physician in diagnosis and treatment. The organic acid test is the most sensitive test for damage to mitochondrial energy production. The organic acid test provides a snapshot of a person's nutrient status and metabolism, identifies functional nutritional deficiencies, and identifies specific blocks and metabolic pathways.

These tests look for the damaging effects of many chemicals and also look at markers for damage. Reactive oxygen species and reactive nitrogen species underlie oxidative damage. Elevated reactive species may use up the body's antioxidants, the only protection against cellular and DNA damage. Markers for reactive species include 8-OHdG, lipid peroxidases, p-hydroxyphenylacetate (HPLA), arachidonic acid, and IL-6.

Tests for oxidative damage are:
- Lipid peroxidase for cell wall oxidative damage.
- 8-hydroxy-2'-deoxyguanosine (8-OHdG) testing for DNA oxidative damage.
- Markers for reactive species and antioxidant capacity.

Other screening tests are:
- Porphyrin testing (another functional test for markers of damage).
- Inflammatory markers—hsCRP, TNF alpha, IL-6, AA/EPA, Quinolinate, HPLA.
- Organic acid test.

2. Test for heavy metal toxicity.

To find heavy metals you can test hair, blood, urine, or feces.

The presence and amount of toxic metals may be evaluated a variety of ways, but a chelated urine evaluation for toxic metals is the usual test because it is the most reliable assessment of the body's burden of heavy metals.

Hair analysis used to be used more frequently, but not as much anymore. Hair analysis has the limitation of possible contamination by external sources, such as high minerals or toxins in water, shampoo, soap, hair dyes and other treatments. Also hair analysis may show low readings when the toxic body burden has been sequestered in bone or matrix. Hair analysis may not accurately reflect the *degree* of toxicity or body burden. Although not as reliable as urine tests, hair analysis does have the advantage of being easy and inexpensive.

Blood and urine tests are good to use when someone has had acute exposure. Use blood and urine tests to measure toxicity for someone who has been poisoned, such as a child who swallowed all of the mercury in a thermometer. The mercury would not show up in the hair for weeks. Individual blood tests can be useful to test someone who has been suddenly exposed to a high level of metals.

A chelated or provoked urine sample is the gold standard for heavy metal testing. A chelated six to eight-hour urine collection for essential minerals and toxic metals is the basic test that is ordered to check for the presence of heavy metals. It is the most reliable test to reflect the retention of heavy metals that are stored in the body. It shows your response to a challenge with a chelating agent. The metals are provoked out with a substance like DMSA (meso 2,3-dimercaptosuccinic acid), DMPS (2,3-dimercapto-1-propanesulfonic acid), or EDTA (ethylenediaminetetraacetic acid).

The results are reproducible. The chelated urine test is good for finding out about low levels of multiple metals. We can test before detoxing and after detoxing to see how well we are doing with lowering the heavy metal burden of the body.

To do the test you can do an I.V. chelation with EDTA, take DMPS by injection, or take DMSA or EDTA orally. You then collect all of your urine for 6-24 hours and send a small vial of this urine collection to a good specialty lab. When the results come back, the typical test results will show elevated levels of some of the toxic metals, with lead, cadmium, and mercury most commonly being high.

Traditional physicians rely only on blood levels to diagnose lead toxicity. But the only accurate measurement is a chelated urine test Anti-aging physicians rely on chelated urine samples to evaluate for lead toxicity and evaluate the body burden. But even chelated urine testing can underestimate large body burdens of lead or aluminum because they are bound in bone.

Measure both essential minerals and toxic metals.

The red blood cell mineral analysis is a good test to do before and after chelation. This test is an intracellular mineral analysis that reports on both good minerals as well as the bad heavy metals. The red blood cell mineral analysis measures both essential minerals (good) and toxic metals (bad) to identify your current mineral imbalances and toxic burden for heavy metals.

The red blood cell mineral analysis shows deficiencies of good minerals like magnesium, calcium, and selenium. The red blood cell mineral analysis also shows what tissue levels were over the past four months, the life span of red blood cells.

Test for damage of individual toxic metals.

Now that you have found out the level of each of the metals in your tissues, next you can test to find out how much trouble they are causing. Mercury levels found in quantitative testing do not allow us to determine the damage or safety of the reading. A low level in one person may be causing significant pathology whereas a high reading in another person may not be causing that person any apparent problems.

Urinary porphyrin testing is a measurement of the damage that is currently being caused by specific metals and toxic chemicals. Urinary porphyrin testing is important because it tells us if the toxic metal is causing significant harm to you. Porphyrin tests specifically for damage from these heavy metals: aluminum, arsenic, mercury, and lead. It also tests for damage from these organotoxins: hexachlorobenzene, methylchloride, dioxin, polyvinylchloride, polybrominated biphenyls, and alcohol.

Determine current exposures.

To see if someone is currently being exposed to a toxic metal, many physicians will also order an unprovoked or unchelated test. [203] In the unprovoked test, you test the urine *without* first giving a chelating agent. If the test results come back with a level of a substance that is much greater than lab reference values, it would indicate a current exposure. When this is discovered, the current exposure source should be removed, so that it doesn't continue to contaminate the body.

You may want to do this test before doing the provoked urine test. In the provoked urine test, the chelating agent poses some theoretical risk, because it may push toxic metals into vital organs or may precipitate a serious mineral imbalance if a person already has a mineral imbalance. If an individual wishes to avoid the small risk of complications associated with chelation, an unchelated urine test (6-8 hour) may be analyzed for essential minerals and toxic metals.

The fecal metals test can be done to determine what metals you may be currently ingesting. The fecal metals test isn't a good tool for monitoring levels of heavy metals, because the results are just showing you high levels of metals that you have recently ingested in your food plus the metals that are primarily excreted via the GI tract (like mercury).

3. Test for specific chemical toxins.

We are able to test for the level of specific toxic chemicals or group of chemicals, like chlorinated pesticides and volatile solvents. More and more toxin-specific tests are becoming available each month. If you had a known work exposure to a specific toxin, you would order an analysis for that toxin if that test is available in state-of-the-art testing laboratories. You can test specifically for chlorinated pesticides,[204] DDT, DDE, and the PCB exposure that frequently comes from eating farmed Atlantic salmon.[205]

Solvent testing will spot auto exhaust leaks.[206] Solvents are important to test in people with neurological problems and/or bone marrow issues. Solvents dramatically adversely affect bone marrow. If you have infertility problems, you might order the solvent panel, since solvent toxicity is associated with infertility.

Evidence of damage and history of possible exposure direct this type of testing, as the number of tests for different chemicals is now large and ever-expanding. Specific biochemical abnormalities may also be markers to test for specific toxins.

The most commonly available panels are for:
- Chlorinated pesticides.
- Phthalates and parabens.
- Bisphenol A.
- Polychlorinated-bisphenol (PCBs)
- Organophosphates.
- Volatile solvents.

History of specific exposure is the biggest help a physician can have to guide testing. A work and exposure history leads us into looking for a specific toxin or toxin group that is poisoning you. If your organic acid test shows abnormalities consistent with toxic substances, find out how you are currently being exposed.

The EPA TRI (Toxic Release Inventory) online site is a tremendous resource for patients and physicians to find exposure information. You can look up your zip code, and it will tell you specifically what has been put into the air, water, and land in your area.

You can look up specific companies and manufacturers that are close to you or close to where you work(ed) and see what they are reporting for toxic release into the air, land, and water. There may be a toxic waste company disposing of huge amounts of toxic material from multiple sources in your area. When you see what toxins you are exposed to, it can direct specific testing, so take advantage of this resource and find out what it is that you are being exposed to right now. Get tested for the specific toxins that are being disposed of in your area.

B. SCREEN FOR INFECTIOUS DISEASE OF THE G.I. TRACT.

HEALING GASTROINTESTINAL TRACT PATHOLOGY AND PARASITES REQUIRES STATE-OF-THE-ART TESTING and a knowledgeable physician to interpret the tests, examine the patient, and diagnose and treat the problems.

START WITH THE GUT. Low-grade infections are easily overlooked, especially when depending only on community labs to find infection. Don't expect stool tests done in a hospital or traditional labs to find every infection. Community labs are skilled in finding the serious infections that produce marked disease like Salmonella and Shigella. The organisms that produce "bloody diarrhea" fall into this category.

But to pinpoint the more elusive infections, it is critical to use state-of-the-art labs that specialize in discovering hidden infections. If we don't treat low-grade infection, it becomes a lifelong source of chronic infection with production of toxins on a continuous basis.

Comprehensive GIT profiles.

Get your stool tests sent to a reputable state-of-the-art lab to be evaluated for evidence of infection and poor digestion. If you have even minimal symptoms of GIT dis-ease, get state-of-the-art testing to exclude treatable infection as the source of the disease.

Stool tests done by state-of-the-art laboratories evaluate: digestive function, how well fats, proteins, carbohydrates and other nutrients are absorbed in the ileum, presence of yeast or bacterial infections, dysbiosis (imbalance in intestinal bacteria), parasitic infection and other indicators of digestive dysfunction. It may cost you $150 to $400 out of your pocket, but the alternative could be thousands of dollars and loss of health through a mistaken diagnosis. More serious disease warrants full state-of-the-art GIT testing. DrHormone.org will give you more information about the stool tests that are required to discover intestinal infections and imbalances.

1. Test for bacterial infections.

There are a number of bacterial infections that can be quite asymptomatic, and it takes a physician's wisdom to know which to treat and which not to treat. Tests often screen for Clostridium difficile, Helicobactor pylori, Campylobacter, and Enterohemorrhagic Esherichia coli (EHEC).

2. Test for viruses.

It is critical to know what virus you have, if it is an active problem right now. Identification might lead to effective treatment that will eradicate the virus. But it is more likely that identification will lead to a diagnosis but not a specific treatment that will help.

Because testing for viruses is often expensive and identifying the virus may not help in any way with treatment, whether or not to test for viruses may be a difficult decision to make. Community labs routinely test for a large number of viruses with sophisticated testing to identify how long the virus has been present and if it is active or not. But your physician's ability to help these viral diseases is quite limited. Often a dreadful disease like Hepatitis C is treated with drugs like interferon, with a great many side effects. The goal is usually to ameliorate a terrible disease state and prolong life. *But the possibility of totally eradicating the disease still falls in the realm of alternative medicine.*

There are specialty labs specializing only in finding stealth viruses, and newer specialty labs have sprung up around Lymes disease. Lymes disease and its associated infections are becoming increasingly common. Specialists in Lymes utilize these specialty labs to understand their patient, diagnose what infections are present, and direct treatments.

3. Test for parasites.

Unfortunately, parasites hide high in the intestines. Many parasites can only be found when the intestinal tract is completely emptied. This requires drinking a laxative and then getting a liquid stool sample many hours later, after many bowel movements have occurred. Your best chance of finding these hard-to-find parasites is to send this last liquid stool sample to a state-of-the-art lab that specializes in finding them. (Some tests don't need purge samples.)

For parasites, community labs only offer ova and parasite exams (O and P), which may lead to incorrect conclusions and waste time and money. O and P is the visual inspection of a tiny portion of the stool. When positive and an organism is identified, the test is very inexpensive and reliable. But when it is negative, it is not helpful because you don't know if you didn't see the organism on the tiny portion of stool examined, or if the organism is not present. This is very dangerous, because it leads the physician and patient to the false belief that they do not have chronic parasitic infection.

You can't find the disease if you don't use the right tests to find it. Traditional MDs and gastroenterologists who follow standard of care say that O and P exam of the stool is adequate, and parasites can be ruled in or out by this exam usually done three times. But in Dr. Swartz's experience, this cursory exam finds only a small fraction of disease. Only a patient who is acutely ill and is shedding large numbers of parasites or ova will have them identified in the O and P exam.

The majority of chronic parasite infections will be missed. The great harm that is done by using community labs to test stool samples is that everyone, including the patient, believes that parasites have been eliminated as a possibility. Therefore testing is not usually repeated. Even if the testing is repeated, when no parasite is found, it is a waste of more money and more time.

Treatment continues for years with great expense and loss of health because of a faulty diagnosis of irritable bowel syndrome, or diverticulitis, or ulcerative colitis. The patient receives expensive medical care that is inappropriate for the actual problem and never recovers his or her health.

In order to pinpoint the problem(s), it is necessary to use specialty labs that offer specific testing for GIT pathology. Specialty labs offer evaluation for parasites, dysbiosis, bacterial pathogens, yeast, digestive function, inflammatory markers, and a lot more. In addition to traditional ova and parasite exam and cultures, specialty labs also offer these tests:

(1) **Antibody testing** at the specialty labs tells you if the organism was present sometime in your body, but not if it is present now.

(2) **Antigens** are parts of an infectious organism and indicate that it is currently present.

(3) **DNA** is the state-of-the-art testing that detects the presence of parasite DNA and can evaluate anaerobic bacteria (95% of the GI flora), which cannot be done with cultures.

Community labs do not offer these antibody tests and only limited antigen tests. None of the testing at community labs can help to answer a more important question, "Is the organism confined to the intestinal tract or disseminated throughout the body?"

Sometimes you need to use a very specific lab or research lab to find systemic activity. "Taenia solium," pork tapeworm, is the most common cause for seizures in Mexico. This disease infects pigs and humans in Asia, Africa, South America, parts of Southern Europe and pockets of North America. Cysts of this pork tapeworm lodge in the brain and are disseminated through the body. *Specialty labs may find antibody present indicating past or present infection, but only research labs or very specific labs that are hard to find test for systemic activity.*

4. Test for yeast.

A stool culture is used to test for yeast. A urine test for D-arabinital is another yeast test available in specialty labs.

Yeast culture test results often include sensitivities. Sensitivities indicate what substances will inhibit the yeast's growth or kill it. Once a patient is predisposed to yeast, it will tend to overgrow again if poor diet and/or antibiotics again support its overgrowth.

5. Test for leaky gut.

To test for leaky gut, drink a solution containing mannitol and lactulose and collect your urine for six hours to be tested. Lactulose (a disaccharide) and mannitol (a monosaccharide) are water-soluble, non-metabolized sugar molecules. The degree of intestinal permeability or malabsorption is reflected in the levels of the two sugars. Mannitol is easily absorbed. Lactulose has larger molecules and is minimally absorbed. If the levels of mannitol and lactulose in the collected urine sample are low, it is indicative of malabsorption. High levels of both molecules indicate leaky gut. High levels of mannitol and low levels of lactulose indicate healthy digestion.

C. TEST HORMONES.

FIRST EVALUATE ADRENALS, THEN INSULIN RESISTANCE, THYROID, SEX HORMONES, GROWTH HORMONE, AND ESTROGEN METABOLISM.

1. Adrenal health testing.

Adrenal health can be measured with a four-point cortisol saliva or blood test. Cortisol levels at 8 am, noon, 5 pm, and 11pm will reveal the diurnal cortisol pattern. It is obviously easier to test saliva than blood. Salivary cortisol testing is well-documented as an accurate assessment. The salivary cortisol test requires filling four test tubes with saliva (not foam)—one around 8 a.m., one at 11 a.m.-noon, one at 4-5 p.m., and one at 11-12 p.m. With a healthy cortisol curve, the first morning tube should be the highest of the day, as it is telling all of the other hormones to wake up for the day. As you adapt to the stresses of the day, the level should come down. The second one should be about two to three times less than the first. If you have good glycemic control, the third should be about even or a tiny bit lower than the second level. The last one should be very low, as now it is time to relax and go to sleep.

Irregular, high elevations of cortisol are probably hypoglycemia. With dysfunctional adrenals, the levels do not mimic this natural curve. Often levels are reversed with higher levels at night. When the curve is reversed, people usually wake exhausted (low cortisol) and in the evening usually feel quite good (high cortisol). In Stage 4 (adrenal exhaustion), cortisol will be continuously low.

Test for cortisol steal by measuring DHEAS. If DHEAS is low, suspect that DHEA is being used up to make cortisol.

2. Insulin resistance testing.

The tests that you will need to get are:

- **Fasting Blood Sugar.** A morning (12-hr) fasting blood glucose will indicate the presence and severity of insulin resistance, but fasting insulin, 2-hour and 3-hour glucose tolerance test or 2-hour or 3-hour postprandial insulin and glucose are further diagnostic guides.
  - o A normal fasting blood sugar is less than 90 mg/dl.
  - o When fasting blood sugar is greater than 90, you are insulin-resistant, and you may be progressing towards type II diabetes.
  - o When blood sugar is less than 81, you are insulin-sensitive, and there is a low risk of diabetes.[207]
- **Hemoglobin A1c (HbA1c)** is a marker for average blood glucose levels over the previous three months. It is a measure of how glycinated your tissues are.
- **Lipids**—Triglycerides.
- **High-sensitivity C-reactive protein.** This test is one measure of the destructive inflammatory response that accompanies metabolic syndrome. This test will tell you more about your heart disease risk than a lipid profile alone.

3. Thyroid health testing.

There are many different ways that the thyroid can malfunction. People may have more than one of these problems at the same time. Clinical symptoms are often more important than test results. Testing is essential and may indicate the source of the symptoms. Thyroid hormones may be suboptimal, and a person may be hypothyroid even with numbers that are in the normal range (subclinical hypothyroidism). Many physicians believe a TSH of 1 is optimal.

TSH is not the best test to measure thyroid function. TSH may not identify peripheral conversion problems, where T4 does not convert to adequate T3. Reference ranges do not reflect if the hormone level is too high or low *for you*. The pituitary may be sluggish (usually with traumatic brain injury) and not increase TSH even though the peripheral tissues need more thyroid hormone.

It is more important to evaluate the free T3 and free T4 levels and bring them into the optimal range. Many physicians prefer direct measurement of hormone levels and order total and free T4, total and free T3, TBG, and RT3.

Autoimmune reactions are a primary cause of thyroid disorders. To diagnose thyroid autoimmunity (Hashimoto's), measure thyroid peroxidase (TPO) antibodies and thyroid-binding globulin (TBG) antibodies. TPO is positive in 85% of cases in Hashimoto's. When there are symptoms of *either* hyperthyroidism or hypothyroidism, screen for thyroid antibodies (TPO and TBG). Also, if antibody tests are positive, screen for gluten allergies with a gliadin antibody test.

You may have Wilson's Temperature Syndrome (WTS) if you typically have a low body temperature. Get a glass thermometer (not battery-operated) and take your temperature several times a day starting three hours after you get up.

If the temperature is consistently below 98.6, you may be able to benefit from treatment for WTS. WTS is characterized by hypothyroid symptoms, low basal body temperature, and normal blood tests. A trial of T3 is diagnostic.

4. Female sex hormone testing.

Begin sex hormone testing if there are symptoms of hormonal deficiency. In women in their active, reproductive years, and those on cyclic BHRT, measure peak estradiol on day 12 and peak progesterone on day 21.

Balance estradiol (E2) and progesterone (P4). If cycling, measure E2 on day 12 and P4 on day 21, and keep them in balance rather than worry about absolute values.

As estrogen levels fluctuate quite a bit, if estrogen is low on the day it is measured, the physician may erroneously prescribe estrogen. This will make everything worse when estrogen is dominant in relation to progesterone. The estrogen dominance may be from the xenoestrogen load which is impossible to measure and/or from estrogen metabolites.

A woman may be estrogen-deficient *and* estrogen-dominant (in relation to progesterone). Absolute levels of estrogen and progesterone are not as important as keeping the two hormones balanced.

Sex hormone testing for women:
- FSH and LH.
- Estradiol.
- Progesterone
- Testosterone.
- DHEA-S.
- Estrogen metabolism.

5. Male sex hormone testing.
To check sex hormone levels in men, draw serum:
- Total and free testosterone.
- Total estrogen.
- LH.
- DHEA-S.
- In men with erectile dysfunction and in all older males, add PSA and prolactin.
- Estrogen metabolism.

6. Human Growth Hormone testing.
Human Growth Hormone (HGH) levels fluctuate very rapidly. Optimization of growth hormone (GH) first involves evaluating the GH status of the individual. The majority of physicians just order a blood test for IGF-1. GH fluctuates so rapidly that attempts to measure it are of little help in establishing the over-all adequacy of GH. IGF-1 is the product of GH produced by the liver that actually mediates the GH effect on the body, and it is a very stable value. Some physicians still measure urinary GH levels, but a single blood draw is more convenient than a timed urine sample. Human Growth Hormone replacement must be monitored. The tests that you will need are:
- A serum IGF-1, (Insulin-like Growth Factor 1) or Urine GH.[208]
- IGFBP3 (Insulin-like Growth Factor Binding Protein 3).

7. Estrogen metabolism testing.
Optimizing estrogen metabolism is important for both men and women, especially so for women who are taking supplemental estrogen in any form. Even if you are not taking supplemental estrogen, correcting harmful estrogen metabolism is necessary if you want to decrease your risk of cancer.[209] Everyone produces some estrogen (even men), and we are all exposed to estrogen-mimicking substances in our environment in the form of plastics, pesticides, herbicides, and other chemicals.

When you go to a doctor, he or she will usually insist on the standard tests to see if you have cancer. But very few doctors look at how well you are detoxifying all of the hormones and chemicals you are ingesting from your environment. 90-95% of all cancer is related to environment and lifestyle.[210]

Doctors who ignore estrogen metabolism (and that includes almost all doctors everywhere) do not understand the importance of abnormal estrogen metabolism. Even if you have been born with genes that make it more likely that you will get cancer, if you supply the liver with the enzymes and other nutrients needed for good estrogen metabolism and have a healthy lifestyle, you can greatly reduce the likelihood of those genes expressing themselves to cause cancer and other diseases.

Every man and woman should get an estrogen metabolism test. An important step to take to prevent cancer is to get an estrogen metabolism test and then to correct faulty estrogen metabolism by adding certain foods and supplements. It is important that both men and women be tested.

Whether or not you are using any kind of HRT, you need to find out if you are metabolizing your estrogen primarily down a good, bad, or ugly pathway and if you are methylating well. *This is not optional for anti-aging medicine, because xenoestrogens are causing bad and ugly estrogen metabolism in the majority of us.*

You can't safely replace deficient estrogen without doing this test. The only safe way to replace deficient estrogen is to measure how it is being metabolized by getting an estrogen metabolism test and to correct abnormal metabolism.

D. CHECK MARKERS FOR INFLAMMATION.

- *IF YOU HAVE A LOT OF INFLAMMATORY SYMPTOMS,* you can get tested for the inflammatory chemicals elaborated by belly fat (**TNF-alpha, IL-6**).
- **Get a high sensitivity CRP (called hs-CRP or cardiac CRP).** C-reactive protein is produced by the liver. CRP rises when there is silent inflammation throughout the body. Regular CRP is not the same as hs-CRP.
- **Measure the ratio of arachidonic acid (AA) to eicosapentaenoic acid (EPA) in plasma** to measure the proinflammatory state. This helps to identify the risk of heart disease and other chronic and inflammatory processes.
- **Homocysteine** is a naturally occurring amino acid found in blood plasma. High levels of homocysteine are believed to increase the chance of heart disease,[211] stroke,[212] Alzheimer's disease,[213] and osteoporosis.[214] Homocysteine is increased by methylation defects.

E. CHECK NEUROTRANSMITTER LEVELS.

NEUROTRANSMITTERS ARE BEST ASSESSED CLINICALLY. The best overall assessment of brain neurotransmitter levels is to take an inventory of deficiency symptoms for neurotransmitters.

- The gold standard for testing neurotransmitters in the brain is to test the levels in the cerebral spinal fluid (CSF). Blood platelet levels are equal to CSF levels.
- Neurotransmitter levels in blood and urine may be influenced on a moment-to-moment basis by diet, activity level, sleep patterns, stress, and a number of other factors and do not correlate with CSF levels. The majority of serotonin is from the G.I. tract, so urinary values don't necessarily reflect what is happening in the brain.
- An accurate assessment of neurotransmitter levels may be made by testing neurotransmitter precursors and metabolites with organic acid tests, amino acid plasma tests, and RBC mineral analysis. The organic acid test reveals vitamin and cofactor deficiencies that block metabolic pathways. Amino acid precursors may not help neurotransmitter deficiencies if the vitamins and cofactors are deficient.
- Kynurenate and quinolinate are good markers to check for neurological inflammation.
- Neurotransmitters have a very complex interrelationship, and you must know the state of each neurotransmitter to successfully balance them.
- To optimize hormones, accurate neurotransmitter testing is required. To optimize neurotransmitters, accurate hormone testing is required.

Step III. INDIVIDUALIZE TREATMENT PLANS.

AFTER RECEIVING YOUR TEST RESULTS, take them to an anti-aging or alternative, functional medical physician who will understand the test results and who will be able to diagnose and treat you. These forward-thinking physicians will treat mild or moderate hormone imbalances and can guide you in correcting the sick metabolism caused by toxicity, infection, and hormone imbalance that makes it impossible to lose weight and enjoy health.

Do one thing at a time, and evaluate the results before making another intervention. Now that you have your test results, under your physician's guidance you can use the results of your testing to improve your health dramatically one step at a time.

If you do more than one thing at a time, you can't understand what is doing what. Your physician will prioritize your treatment and separate it so that you can see what makes you feel good or bad.

A. TREAT TOXICITY.

HOW CAN WE STAY HEALTHY if we are choking off our blood vessels with toxins that are scraping and burning their way through us? How can we stay healthy if our cell membranes and our mitochondria are being damaged by metals and chemicals?

Instead of a crisis-management mentality, we *all* need to approach the problem proactively. Instead of waiting until our health deteriorates to a degree where we are seriously ill, we need to take steps right now, no matter how sick we are, to identify and remove the toxic burden. We need to do everything we can to remove these toxic substances from our bodies. In most cases, fat-soluble environmental toxins cannot be excreted easily without our diligence. These toxins remain in our tissues until we take steps to remove them. Until we remove this toxicity from our bodies, it is impossible to normalize our weight, balance our hormones, and enjoy the health that should be our birthright.

Remove heavy metals and chemicals even if levels are low, because *any* amount of these toxins is damaging our health, right down to the cellular level of the tiniest capillary. Even if you find out that you only have low levels of toxins, you are not safe from their damage. Low levels are stored in the body and accumulate.[215] As time goes on, low levels get higher and higher because they are so fat-soluble and not easily removed from the body. Toxins burn cell membranes and scratch the lining of your blood vessels. Toxins damage the mitochondria (the powerhouses of the cells). Even small degrees of toxicity cause poorer functioning of every organ, including eyes, skin, heart; you name it, because you have blood vessels in every tissue and organ.

We are all filled with heavy metals and toxic chemicals.[216] We are able to eliminate tiny amounts that grow out in the hair and nails. You may pass some out in your stools. Because there is no easy way to eliminate them, we all accumulate metals and chemical toxins. Because our environment is so permeated with these metals and chemicals, we must get aggressive in eliminating them from our bodies if we want to return to health. We can reduce our risks of all disease, especially heart disease and cancer, by removing as much of these metals and chemicals as we can. You can get these toxins out, but it takes work on your part.

When you get metals and toxic chemicals into you, you will continue to have them inside you until you take action to chelate them out and detoxify them. Don't try to do it too quickly, but do continue to detox heavy metals for the rest of your life.

Your secret action plan to remove toxicity:
- **Don't take toxins in.**
- **Open the channels of elimination.**
- **Eliminate toxins with specific treatments.**

1. Don't take in the poisons.

If you don't put toxins in, you don't have to work to get them out.

Air:
- **Get a good high-quality air filter for your home.**
- **Get a furnace inspection** and tune-up before using the furnace each year. Check gas appliances to make sure that they are properly vented to avoid breathing in carbon monoxide. Use a carbon monoxide detector in boat cabins and in your home. If it has a reading above 10 ppm, find the source and eliminate it.
- **Check for radon** if you live in a radon-prone area. Take steps to remove it if you find it.
- **If you have a moisture problem in your home, find the source of the moisture and eliminate it.** Remove water-damaged materials. Allergies to mold are serious health problems. Use a dehumidifier if you live in a humid area.
- **Never store gasoline or volatile solvents** in basements or attached garages where fumes can leak into the house.

Water:
- **Drink purified water.** Use a good water filtration system and change the filters frequently or buy reverse osmosis water. Supplement with essential elements like magnesium and trace minerals that have been removed in the purification process. When you leave your home, take that purified water with you in your BPA-free water bottle, so that you avoid drinking tap water when you are away from home.
- **If you have a well, it may be contaminated.** Make sure that you have tested the water. Check the TRI report for the chemicals in your area.
- **Stop ingesting halides** (chlorine, fluorine, bromine). Filter your water and use natural toothpaste without fluoride. Avoid chlorinated and brominated pools.

Food:
The agricultural practices involving the use of multiple toxins on an industrial level are major contributors to our toxic food supply.[217] Vegetarians and those of us who eat more live foods have lower toxin levels.[218] [219]
- **Stop eating all canned, refined, and processed food.** These foods are dead and polluted. They have no life vitality. The canning process adds chemicals.[220] [221] The refining process removes valuable nutrients and adds more toxic chemicals. Frozen food, though not as good as fresh, is OK, as it retains much of the life vitality of the food if it has not been processed and lacks the preservatives and toxins. Read the labels and avoid buying anything with nitrites,[222] hydrogenated oils,[223] trans fats,[224] and preservatives.
- **When buying meat, fish, and fowl, get it as fresh as possible and organic.** Don't eat U.S. beef that is not organic when organic alternatives are available. If it does not say that it was raised without antibiotics and/or hormones, don't buy it if you can find alternatives without antibiotics or hormones. Only eat organic chicken.
- **Avoid farmed fish and shellfish and eat smaller ocean fish.**

- *Avoid trans-fatty acids (hydrogenated vegetable oils).*
- *Avoid sugar and artificial sweeteners.*
- *Eat organic food.* Although organic foods are not completely free of toxins, they are less toxic than non-organic foods and have higher levels of nutrients.[225] Eating organic food is, in general, a better choice than eating non-organic food, especially for those foods that are notorious for their toxicity because they are heavily sprayed with chemicals. If fruits and vegetables are not organic, only eat with those with a skin that you can peel off, and don't eat the skin. Buying organic food does not necessarily guarantee that you are getting anything different from the cheaper, non-organic food. Sometimes, the only thing different about the food is the packaging. You don't need to be as concerned about buying non-organic foods that are not sprayed as heavily. For example, broccoli is one of the least toxic vegetables. Buying non-organic broccoli causes little toxicity.
- *Grow your own organic garden* to assure that the produce that you are consuming is free of toxic herbicides, pesticides, and artificial fertilizers. Sprouting in jars is a great way to get fresh greens.[226] By enriching your garden soil with your compost, you can grow your own food that will nourish your body with the vitamins and minerals that are needed to ensure health. Concentrate your efforts on growing healthy food for your family
- *Don't consume non-organic dairy products that contain growth hormone.*
- *Minimize your consumption of GMO food* by avoiding beets, wheat, canola, soybeans, and corn of any kind. Instead of canola oil, use olive oil. For carbohydrates, concentrate on brown rice, quinoa, millet, and starchy veggies.
- *Avoid eating the 12 most toxic fruits and vegetables.* If the food is on the Environmental Working Group's DIRTY DOZEN list, buy it organic or don't buy it. [227]

The "Dirty Dozen" (starting with the worst):
1. Apples.
2. Celery.
3. Sweet bell peppers.
4. Peaches.
5. Strawberries.
6. Nectarines (imported).
7. Grapes (imported).
8. Spinach.
9. Lettuce.
10. Cucumbers.
11. Blueberries (domestic).
12. Potatoes.

These foods are usually safe even without being labeled as organic. "Cleanest 12" (starting with the best):
1. Onions.
2. Sweet corn (frozen).
3. Pineapples.
4. Avocados.
5. Cabbage.
6. Sweet peas (frozen).
7. Asparagus.
8. Mangoes.
9. Eggplant.
10. Kiwi fruit.
11. Cantaloupe.
12. Sweet potatoes.

Drugs:

- *Quit using toxic stimulants:* caffeine, tobacco, diet sodas, regular sodas, diet pills, and alcohol.
- *Give up all unnecessary pharmaceuticals and synthetic hormones.* Taking Tylenol (acetaminophen) is a bad thing to do to your liver. NSAIDs (ibuprofen, naproxen) are a bad thing to do to your body.
- *Don't smoke.*

Electromagnetic Radiation:

- *Don't live near high voltage power lines* on big steel towers. These huge power lines are very disruptive to health.
- *Connect electrical devices in your bedroom to power strips and turn them off* before you go to sleep. Don't sleep with your head near any outlets.
- *Keep your cell phone far from your bed.*

Chemicals:

- *Avoid using harsh chemicals* of any kind. Find safer alternatives. Use only mild disinfectants and soaps. Use only "green" products.
- *Don't use pesticides or herbicides.* Don't spray your home with insecticides. Use baits to kill insects (keep away from children) and seal off insects' entrances into your home. Desiccants like diatomaceous earth and silica aerogel are helpful.
- *If you must use dry cleaned clothes,* air out your clothes outside before wearing them.
- *If you must buy a new car,* roll the windows down to air it out for several days before using it.
- *Try to avoid living in an area where toxic chemicals are used.* One of the worst places is downwind of any coal-burning power plant, because mercury is a by-product. Coal is a foremost reason for environmental contamination all over the planet.
- *Avoid spray cleaners,* so that you don't aerosolize the poisons that can harm eyes, lungs, and skin. Use powders or liquid.
- *Thoroughly air out a home that has been recently painted.*
- *Don't use varnish or wax in enclosed spaces.*
- *Don't use mothballs.* Cedar chips are effective against moths.
- *Avoid using personal care products with chemicals.* Use natural alternatives like coconut oil for your skin. Instead of bathing in toxic chemicals like bubble bath, use Epsom salts and/or baking soda, which are excellent detoxification baths. Underarm deodorants and most skin lotions are toxic. Don't use them. Makeup is a huge source of toxicity for women. Avoid facial peels. Avoid cosmetics, deodorants, unnatural shampoos, fluoridated toothpaste, processed food, and beer. Only use non-pesticidal lice shampoos that use enzymes to kill lice and their eggs. Avoid plastics, dry-cleaning, after-shave lotion, nail polish, nail polish remover, hair spray, and DEET-based insect repellants. Don't drink out of plastic water bottles. Infants chewing on plastic toys, teething rings, and pacifiers are ingesting phthalates.
- *Avoid being around new wood, furniture, and carpets* until they have off-gassed these chemicals.
- *Do not use pet shampoos or flea collars.*
- *Avoid living in a chlordane-treated home.* If you do live in a chlordane-treated home, don't disturb the soil around the foundation.
- *Avoid the use of Teflon* non-stick pans, Gore-Tex clothing, and coated cardboard restaurant leftover containers.
- *Avoid the use of Styrofoam.*
- *Avoid using pottery bowls and mugs* made in small shops, especially from other countries, as they may have lead glazes that will leech into your food and drink.
- *Avoid using crystal glassware* that contains lead or glassware that is carved and shiny.

- *To avoid BPA, avoid using plastic containers for food storage if they have the number 3 or 7 recycling mark on the bottom.* Especially don't microwave these plastics. It is better not to microwave at all for that matter, as you are killing the enzymes in your food and sending out harmful microwave radiation into the bodies of anyone near the microwave. Use glass bottles and containers. Don't put plastic wrap over food.

Don't put toxic chemicals on your skin.

Whatever we put onto our skin goes directly into our blood. When you put any cosmetics, deodorants, or other products onto your skin, it is as bad as or worse than eating them. When you eat the toxins they go through a first pass through the liver, where some detoxification occurs. But when you put the chemicals onto your skin, most toxic chemicals are absorbed through your skin and go directly into your blood, without the first pass through the liver.

Avoid the use of sunscreens with toxic chemicals like parabens, nanoparticles, and oxybenzone. We can use natural alternatives, cover ourselves, limit our sun exposure,[228] and stay out of the sun during peak exposure periods of 10 a.m. to 2 p.m. This is especially important during summer months and at latitudes closer to the equator.

Don't stay out in the sun thinking that your sunscreen will protect you from skin cancer.[229] It may well not. "When the Environmental Working Group (EWG) analyzed 783 sunscreens, the group determined that only 16% of sunscreens on the market are both safe and effective."

Avoid using anything with titanium dioxide in it. Because manufacturers are not required to tell you if nanoparticles are present or not, it is best to use only natural products. U.S. sunscreen makers are not required to list oxybenzone either.

There *are* natural sunscreens with no harmful chemicals in them. Don't forget good old zinc oxide. It may look funny, but it does offer protection, is somewhat water-resistant, and is not harmful.

Metals

- *Because of multiple dangers inherent in the use of chelating agents, your physician should guide you in chelation therapy.* There are concerns about single-dose chelating agents redistributing the toxins into more sensitive areas. Also, all chelating agents bind necessary minerals as well as toxic ones. Serious, even fatal, mineral imbalances may occur with chelating agents. Long-term use of natural non-prescription chelating agents, like NAC and chlorella, are safe and effective for low-level toxicity.
- *Limit intake of cadmium.* Eat organic foods, don't smoke, and get adequate zinc.
- *Limit aluminum intake.* Don't use antiperspirants and deodorants. Instead bathe frequently to remove odor-causing bacteria from the skin. Use natural soaps like Dr. Bronner's. Don't use aluminum-containing antacids, cosmetics, or aluminum cookware. Filter your water with a good, high-quality water filtration system.
- *Remove mercury fillings (amalgams).* Stop eating mercury-containing foods such as tuna and other large fish. Avoid injectable vaccines that contain mercury (thimerosol).
- *Use untreated wood.*
- *Avoid the use of copper cooking utensils.*

Protect yourself from toxic chemicals.

Glutathione will help to protect you from toxic chemicals. Many heavy metals and toxic chemicals do their damage primarily by formation of free radicals--reactive oxygen species (ROS) and reactive nitrogen species (RNS). ROS and RNS produce oxidative damage to the cell membranes and DNA. Glutathione is the primary means the body has of eliminating free radicals. Most of these chemicals will detoxify faster in the presence of glutathione.[230]

Oral liposomal glutathione will not be destroyed through the digestive process. Glycine is also very useful. N-acetyl-cysteine (NAC) is an inexpensive oral supplement that will increase glutathione and acts as a heavy metal chelator.

Detox with diet.

Reduce the fat-soluble toxic burden by eating brown rice, rice bran fiber, chlorophyll, and drinking green tea. Some substances will help to remove toxicity. Eat cilantro, chlorella, and high doses of Vitamin C.[231] EAT LIVE FOODS, not dead things. Avoid all processed foods. Eat lots of organic fruits and vegetables. Make salads. For dressings, make your own with flax oil or olive oil. Do not use restaurant or store-bought salad dressings.

Detox with homeopathics.

Homeopathics have no reported adverse reactions and do not affect regular allopathic (prescription drugs) medications. They act on a completely different level, but they may produce unpleasant effects as they help and heal. *Seeing a physician to guide you is essential for successful treatment.* They are effective, safe, and easy.

2. Open elimination channels.

It is important to cleanse the liver, gall bladder, intestines, and skin before and during fat loss. Cleanse the organs of elimination in the order given to get the best results.

First, Cleanse the Large Intestine.

The large intestine is the primary organ of cleansing and detoxification. Help your large intestine along by eating lots of natural fiber, by taking supplemental fiber (psyllium, pectin, and/or other natural fibers), and bentonite. Be careful. If diseases are too advanced, fiber may be very irritating.

Increasing fiber intake has many health benefits.[232] [233] Fiber helps to remove excess estrogen from the bodies of both men and women, reducing cancer risk.[234] Other advantages of taking fiber include treating constipation, colon cancer prevention, balancing female sex hormones, and prevention of hemorrhoids. There are many brands on the market. Avoid any with sugar, artificial sweeteners, or preservatives. Read the labels carefully. Many of them are toxic and defeat the purpose of using them.

Bentonite clay is a natural cleanser that may be added to fiber to bind toxins until they can be excreted.[235] Bentonite, like activated charcoal, will adsorb (bind) anything. It will bind medication as avidly as toxins, so take it one hour before medications or one half hour after medications. If you find it constipating, decrease the dose.

Colonic cleansers, colonics, and enemas are a great way to detoxify,[236] even removing heavy metals. Colonic cleansers are supplements taken to decrease the time that stool remains in the colon, cleansing the colon every 24 hours. This gives your body less time to absorb toxic compounds that are sitting there. "Perfect 7" is a fiber cleanser that contains herbs and bentonite.

Colonics are a mechanical means of deep colon cleansing. This requires professional equipment and a colon therapist. Colonics may be one of the most effective ways of deep cleansing.

Enemas utilize a gravity-fed enema/douche bag and are extremely useful for a home program of detoxification. Coffee enemas are the mainstay of successful cancer therapies, like the Gerson therapy.

Second, Cleanse the Liver

Pay attention to liver detoxification, in order to excrete the harmful toxins safely as they are released into the blood stream. Regular liver (hepatic) detoxification removes the toxicity that results from our exposure to xenoestrogens, pharmaceuticals, and all of the toxicity that we are ingesting from our environment.

If you have serious health issues such as chronic fatigue and fibromyalgia, be careful with liver detoxification at first. Detoxify the liver only under your doctor's supervision. The body must be prepared to throw off the toxins. People may become even sicker when they begin to detoxify these dangerous substances if they do not have the energy reserves to get rid of the poisons, or if they overwhelm the organs of elimination. Kidneys are especially vulnerable to injury.

Coffee enemas are a most important liver detoxification tool. Coffee enemas are major components of many treatment programs for degenerative diseases such as arthritis and diabetes. Take coffee enemas regularly to cleanse the liver and intestines of toxicity. Coffee enemas are easy to do, and you can do them at home.

Coffee enemas became established into medicine when Dr. Max Gerson began using them to treat cancer patients in the 1930's.[237] Substances in coffee detoxify carcinogens by neutralizing free radicals.[238] Most proponents believe that the major value of the coffee enema is that a coffee enema retained for fifteen minutes will cause the liver to dump its toxic load. Coffee enemas are stimulating, so don't do them late in the day or they may make sleep difficult. The coffee is absorbed directly into the bloodstream, where it is carried to the liver and gall bladder. The coffee stimulates the liver and gallbladder to dump toxins into the lumen of the intestines, where they can be excreted from the body. Taking organic chlorella an hour before the coffee enema will help bind toxic substances in the bile, so that they can be eliminated.[239 240 241]

When doing any kind of enema, *it is important to minimize the risks* involved by using liquid that is no warmer than room temperature, sterilizing equipment, and never sharing equipment. Never use tap water that has not been boiled or filtered. The intestines may easily be contaminated with bacteria, viruses, and parasites from water. Lube the tip to avoid tearing anal tissue.

To take a coffee enema, begin by using only a small amount of coffee (a half teaspoon) in a 12-cup coffee maker. You may work up to three tablespoons of coffee if it doesn't irritate the intestines and isn't too stimulating. Prop up the hips with towel-covered pillows placed next to the toilet. Allow the liquid to run in slowly, a cup at a time, until you feel full. To move the enema through the colon, you may start on the left side, turn to your back, and then go to the right side, then back on the left, all the while massaging your belly to loosen waste. Try to hold the mixture as long as possible. Some people will only be able to manage a few seconds. Others may be able to hold it longer. Fifteen minutes is ideal. Don't worry if you can't hold it for a long time.

You may follow the coffee mixture with plain water to rinse out the coffee. A second enema four to six hours after the first can greatly speed the exit of toxins pulled out during the first enema. Adding magnesium (Epsom salts) may improve the results.

Support both phases of liver detoxification.

The liver has a system of enzyme detoxification that will remove the toxins, if it is supplied with all of the nutrients to make it work properly. Fat-soluble toxins have to be metabolized in the liver into water-soluble chemicals and then excreted through the large intestine, skin, or kidneys.

When liver health is not good, the liver cannot turn the fat-soluble toxins into water-soluble toxins. They will stay inside the body, adding to oxidative stress and disease.

There are two major phases of liver detoxification, Phase I and Phase II. Our liver detoxification system is the most effective defense we have against xenoestrogens, steroids, prescription and non-prescription drugs, alcohol, and all manner of toxins absorbed from the environment. Many of these toxins are fat-soluble, which make them require both Phase I and Phase II detoxification to be eliminated. Proper Phase I and Phase II detoxification in the liver and bowels is also crucial to metabolize our hormones.

THE LIVER MUST BE SUPPLIED WITH ALL OF THE NUTRIENTS NEEDED FOR BOTH OF THESE PHASES TO WORK, OR ELSE IT WILL NOT DETOXIFY AT ALL.

In Phase I, fat-soluble substances are converted into more dangerous intermediate compounds. During this step, the liver hydroxylates the toxins into dangerous free radicals. These free radicals may destroy proteins, specifically the DNA inside the nucleus of the cells. This is called oxidative stress.

Phase II of the detox cycle makes the intermediate substances water-soluble so that they can be eliminated. In Phase II, the liver takes the dangerous free radicals that were produced in Phase I and conjugates them with other substances making them water-soluble, so that they can be eliminated safely through the urine, sweat, bile, and feces.

Phase I may be highly toxic if not supported by Phase II. Cigarette smoke and charbroiled meats are dangerous because they may cause the Phase I system to kick in but not the Phase II system (more so in genetically-susceptible individuals).[242] [243]

It is important to provide ample antioxidants during detoxification to avoid free radical damage.[244] It is important to be ready to neutralize these toxic substances as they become liberated from the tissues. If you decide to do a liver detox and you support only the Phase I detox system without having the nutrients that support the Phase II system, you will be producing more free radicals without having anything to neutralize and excrete them.

Don't cut corners in order to save money. The only safe way to detoxify the body is to provide *all* of the nutrients necessary to run both phases of liver detoxification.

Metagenics, Thorne, Xymogen, and other companies have developed specific supplements to support both Phase I and II detoxification cycles. Once the toxins are processed by the liver, then a clean and open pathway via the large intestine or skin will cleanse the body of its poisons.

For Phase II to work properly, you require co-factors from the diet. If you have a poor diet, you will not have proper Phase II detoxification. *Vitamins and minerals are co-factors that are necessary for metabolic enzymes to function.* If co-factors have been depleted and are not resupplied regularly, Phase II detoxification will be inhibited.

Vitamins C and E and glutathione are antioxidants that scavenge free radicals, turning them into safe metabolites. If you run out of sulfur-containing amino acids or selenium, Phase I will continue to produce free radicals, but Phase II will not run. These free radicals may lead to cancer and other degenerative diseases.[245]

Flavonoids are particularly important as co-factors to ensure adequate Phase II detoxification.[246] One of these flavonoids is ellagic acid. It will induce several Phase II enzymes. It can be found in red grapes or green tea. Other foods that contain compounds that will induce Phase II enzyme activity include garlic, Brussels sprouts, rosemary, quercetin, rutin, hesperidin, and cabbage.

Also take glycine, N-Acetyl Cysteine (NAC), and methyl B-12. Methylation is an important part of the Phase II reaction.

Methyl B-12 supplies the "methyl" in the methylation. The sublingual form is the most effective way to take it orally. Other methyl donors are DMG (dimethylglycine), TMG (trimethylglycine), 5-MTHF (5-methyltetrahydrofolate), and MSM (methylsulfonylmethane).

Use activated Folic acid (5MTHF). Folic acid is needed for methylation to occur. But sometimes people can't break down ordinary folic acid. For this reason, it is wise to supplement with the activated form of folic acid, called 5MTHF, or 5-methylyetrahydrofolate.

There is a Phase III system also. Phase III is bile salt excretion and enterohepatic reuptake of bile salts in the ileum. This is important in heavy metal detoxification.

Mercury is excreted in the bile salts and re-absorbed in the ileum. If you take cilantro, which mobilizes mercury, it will be re-absorbed in the ileum if you don't take chlorella or bentonite to bind it.

Take these Nutrients to support Phase I detoxification:
- B vitamins. Riboflavin (B-2). Pyridoxine (B-6). Methyl B-12. Niacin (B-3).
- Folic Acid.
- Glutathione.
- Branched chain amino acids.
- Vitamin C, E, N-Acetyl-Cysteine (NAC), Alpha-Lipoic Acid (ALA).
- Carotenoids—beta-carotene, lycopene, lutein.
- Bioflavonoids.
- Beets, berries, grapes (anthocyanadins).
- Pomegranate, strawberries, raspberries, walnuts (ellagic acid).
- Green tea catechins (polyphenols).
- Fruit and vegetable skin (quercetin).

Take Phase II detoxification nutrients:
- Minerals (zinc, selenium, magnesium).
- Amino acid replacement (especially sulfur-containing amino acids).
- Flavonoids – ellagic acid and green tea catechins.
- Glucosinolates – Cruciferous vegetables and alliums like onions and garlic.
- Monoterpenes (citrus peel, cherries).
- Silymarin (milk thistle).
- ALA and NAC to remove metals and free radicals.
- MSM – Methylsulfonylmethane as a sulfur source.
- Glycine to remove chemicals in the liver.
- Magnesium glycinate.
- Malic acid. Magnesium malate dissolves bile salts, especially with orthophosphoric acid.
- Calcium D-glucarate increases estrogen metabolism and xenoestrogen clearance.

Take Supplements that support both Phase I and Phase II detoxification:
- Vitamin D.
- Zinc.
- Selenium.
- EPAs.
- Methylation support–B-6, activated folate, methyl B-12, tri-methyl glycine (TMG).
- Antioxidant support (Vitamins A, C, and E, ALA, protein, milk thistle, green tea, NAC).

Mobilize the Lymphatic System

MOBILIZE THE LYMPH to get rid of edema and remove toxins stored in the fat. People feel better and they sleep better. Anything that stimulates the lymphatic system to carry off toxicity is good. There are twelve quarts of lymph in the body. It is the only irrigation source for nutrients, including minerals, to get to the cells. So it is extremely important to keep the lymph moving to nourish the cells.

Six things you can do to mobilize the lymph system:
1. **Exercise** is essential. It is the best form of lymph massage and drainage. If you can't go to the gym, do exercises at home. Add more exercise by parking farther away. Whatever you can do to exercise, just do it.
2. **Lymphatic massage** is great. The lymph system does not have its own pump. Toxins in the body cause sluggishness and a general lack of energy.

3. **Baths.** Epsom salts and baking soda baths are easy and effective. There are many specialty bathing salts that are excellent alternatives to Epsom salt.
4. **Dry-brush massage.** This moves the surface lymph which is the most stagnant portion of the lymph system. The brushes used in dry-brush massage have a certain stiffness of bristles to move the lymph without injuring the skin. Always brush toward the heart.
5. **Lymph draining and wraps.** Professionals in hospitals trained in lymphatic drainage use special massage and wraps to treat the serious lymphedema that follows surgical procedures like lymph node removal for breast cancer. It can be used very effectively for edema in the legs. You place an elastic wrap starting at the foot and moving up the leg in conjunction with elevation. Whenever mobilizing large amounts of toxic lymphedema, it is important to have the channels of elimination open.
6. **Saunas.** Far-infrared (FIR) sauna is the best because it heats deep into the tissues to remove toxicity.

Detox Through the Skin.

USE A SAUNA to sweat out toxins stored in fat.[247] [248] This is a great way to eliminate dioxin and all other toxins.

A portable, collapsible far-infrared sauna (FIR) is a comfortable way to detox, as your head sticks out through the top. The FIR sauna is much more comfortable than regular saunas or steam rooms. The other saunas may be difficult to tolerate, especially for those with respiratory problems. Your body gently heats up in the FIR sauna.

You can buy a portable FIR sauna with arm holes so that you can read or work on your computer. A hole in the top allows your head to stick out. With your head remaining cool, you can tolerate the heat on the rest of your body enough to really get a good sweat going. With openings for your arms, you can read or type while sitting in the sauna for several hours each day. You may have to let the sauna air out (outgas) before using it.

The FIR sauna is more effective than regular saunas, as the FIR rays penetrate directly into the fat stores to mobilize the toxins and sweat them out. Another advantage over the saunas at your local gym is that you won't be breathing in the toxicities that are being eliminated by other sauna users. FIR saunas help the body to increase the toxic content of sweat by 5-15%. FIR saunas help with increasing circulation.[249] [250] You will detox faster when you keep at it repeatedly. After taking a FIR sauna, it is important to shower well, cleansing the toxins off the skin. Pregnant women should avoid saunas.

FIR saunas help with chronic health problems. The FIR sauna has been shown to reduce musculoskeletal pain like back pain and neck pain.[251] Insomnia and depression also decrease with increased use of the FIR sauna.[252] FIR saunas particularly help people with auto-immunity, fibromyalgia,[253] rheumatoid arthritis, and chronic fatigue. [254] [255] [256]

Mobilize Toxins From the Matrix.

Only after thoroughly cleansing the large intestine, liver, lymphatics, and skin do we concern ourselves with mobilizing the toxins out of the matrix. Before mobilizing toxins from the matrix, cleanse intestines, liver, and skin, and support the detox cycles of the liver to open the channels of elimination.

The matrix is the space outside your cells and between the capillary bed and the cell. This space is the storage dump for toxins. These toxins are deposited here to keep them out of vital organs like your brain, and kidneys. It is dangerous to try to mobilize these toxins out of the matrix if the liver, intestines, and skin are not prepared to remove them from the body. If the liver, intestines, and skin can't immediately remove toxins that have been mobilized from the matrix, the toxins could end up in vital organs where they can do serious damage.

Fasting is one of the fastest ways to mobilize toxins out of the matrix. Fasting, by complete abstinence from food, is the quickest and most dangerous way to mobilize toxins from the matrix. When well-tolerated, fasting may lower risk for metabolic and cardiovascular disease.[257] *But, if done incorrectly, fasting may be hazardous or even fatal.*

Electrolyte imbalances may occur and may be fatal. Consulting experts in how to fast safely is essential. If you decide to fast, do it only under professional supervision until you learn to do it well. *It is necessary to cleanse the colon when fasting,* in order to quickly remove toxins that are deposited into the intestines (bentonite and coffee enemas). Short fruit fasts for one to three days, eating only non-acidic fruit, such as apples, watermelon, or mangos are the safest and easiest way to start.

If you have weakened adrenals, blood sugar issues, or thyroid problems, do not fast. Fasting may lead to hypothyroidism by blocking the conversion of T4 to the active T3 hormone (Wilson's Temperature Syndrome). Fasting stresses the adrenals and should be avoided with Stage 3-4 dysfunction. Hypoglycemia may occur during fasting, especially if you are prediabetic or diabetic. Always carry juice with you and drink it if you feel a blood sugar drop (cold sweat, faint, stomach ache, heart pounding).

Certain homeopathic remedies help to mobilize toxins out of the matrix and into the blood where they can be taken to the organs of elimination and removed from the body. Dr. Reckeweg coined the term, "homotoxicology." His premise is that all disease can be ultimately linked to a toxin in the body. "Heel" is a company that makes homeopathic remedies based on his research and theories. Find a physician who has studied homotoxicology and who will supervise your detoxification and prescribe the remedies that can help you to detox effectively. "Lymphomyosot," a homeopathic made by Heel, effectively mobilizes matrix toxins into the blood. It is so powerful that many patients can't take more than five drops twice a day, or they will become too ill. The Heel detox kit contains "Nux Vomica," to detoxify the intestinal tract, "Berberis Homaccord," to detoxify the urinary tract, and "Lymphomyosot," to mobilize the matrix stores. In cases of severe toxicity, Heel has advanced detox protocols that are very effective adjuncts to other detoxification processes. An added advantage to homeopathics is that they have no interaction with any pharmaceutical drugs, and no allergic reactions have been reported.

Damage occurs when toxins enter the bloodstream: This occurs first when you ingest the poison. You get more damage again when the matrix releases the poison. This is why you may become very ill when you crash diet without immediately taking precautions to remove the toxicity from your body. When undergoing caloric restriction (including the hCG protocol), the body will mobilize toxins out of the matrix and fat and release them into the blood stream. The toxins may become deposited in tissues, like kidney and brain, where they can then damage the organs. This is why dietary programs should be undertaken only with medical supervision and attention given to cleansing the intestines, liver, and skin to avoid poisoning vital organs with toxicity that has been locked up in the matrix for decades.

3. Eliminate heavy metals and chemicals.

After opening all of the organs of elimination, including the large intestine, liver, lymphatic system, skin, and matrix, you can turn your attention to removing heavy metals and chemicals. These metals and chemicals are stored in all of the tissues of the body, but especially in the matrix that surrounds your cells. If you try to remove heavy metals and chemicals before the channels of elimination are open and clear, you may make yourself even sicker and injure brain and kidneys. When toxins are released into the bloodstream, they need to be removed immediately, so that they don't cause damage. If the channels aren't clear, the toxins will be deposited back into the matrix or into organ tissue.

Remove heavy metals with:
- Chelation.
- FIR saunas.
- Bentonite.
- Chlorella and cilantro, NAC, garlic.

Heavy metal poisoning (identified by chelated urine tests) may be treated with chelation until levels are reduced sufficiently. Traditional physicians do not treat low blood levels of heavy metals (no matter what the tissue levels are). They certainly weigh the risks of chelation as greater than the risk of the toxic metal load. *Anti-aging physicians opt for treatment to remove elevated heavy metals.* Treatment of heavy metal toxicity primarily involves chelating agents.

The most effective treatment for heavy metal toxicity is a series of chelation treatments to remove the heavy metals. Before getting chelation, support the organs of detoxification and drainage, especially the kidneys, which are easily damaged in chelation.

The most popular way to remove heavy metals is to use EDTA (ethylenediaminetetraacetic acid). Taking EDTA by any method, I.V., oral, or suppository, is safe under a physician's management. When patients receive chelation, one of the first things that they notice is that they sleep better.

EDTA is a proven chelating agent that has been used for the last seventy years. It has helped many people to overcome many health problems, especially heart disease. It has been proven to be effective and is FDA-approved as an effective treatment for heavy metal poisoning, even for children and the elderly.

Any chelation is dangerous without professional supervision. Chelation binds essential minerals, as well as toxic metals. You may deplete yourself of essential minerals. This is not only dangerous; it may be fatal. Replacement of essential minerals is necessary when using chelators.

EDTA may be used intravenously, orally, and even by suppository. Intravenous is invasive, expensive, time-consuming and very effective. It may cost you hundreds to thousands of dollars to get the thirty I.V.s you need to get these metal levels down significantly. But it is very effective. So if you have the money, the time, and don't mind that needle in your arm, go for the I.V. EDTA chelation. You are getting 100% delivery of the EDTA that way. You may use oral EDTA and EDTA suppositories and get good results also.

The tissue penetration from suppositories, which are held in the rectum for about an hour and a half, has been shown to be about 36%, which is very good for a suppository delivery system. This is because the EDTA dramatically improves the circulation, which is carrying the EDTA to all of the tissues. After the suppository is inserted, blood levels of EDTA rise to a peak, begin to decline, and then rise again to hit two more peaks before finally declining. The enterohepatic circulation keeps the EDTA moving around again and again to increase its effectiveness. Thus the suppositories are longer-acting than the I.V.'s.

DMPS and DMSA are other commonly-used chelators that will grab onto heavy metals so that they can be eliminated from the body. DMSA may be used by injection or orally. DMPS is by injection only. Each has a different affinity for each metal, so your physician can best help you choose the treatment of choice for your condition and plan replacement of essential minerals. Cilantro mobilizes mercury, lead, aluminum, and tin from the brain and spinal cord. Vitamin C also mobilizes mercury stores. After mobilizing it, we can then bind up the mercury with N-acetyl-cysteine (NAC), garlic, MSM, and chlorella so that it can be eliminated. If you take cilantro to mobilize the toxins, make sure you take chlorella to bind the toxins, or the toxins will just be reabsorbed back into the body.

Because chelation will remove the good minerals along with the bad heavy metals, it is essential to take a cell membrane-repairing multi-mineral supplement during chelation. Once your physician has given a course of chelation, he/she will remeasure heavy metals and essential minerals to correct imbalances in essential minerals and direct further treatment of toxic metals.[258]

When you repeat the test again after doing a series of chelations, the results are interesting. Because lead is the metal that is most easily excreted with EDTA, lead levels usually drop after chelation with EDTA. Then aluminum may show up as being really high, even though there wasn't any recent huge exposure to aluminum. What happened is that the aluminum was always there, but the first time the test was done, there was so much mercury and lead binding to the chelator that the binding sites were overwhelmed with the mercury and lead, and the test was unable to accurately detect the other metals.

Lead and aluminum levels may increase, even after chelation. Lead and aluminum that were stored in the bones come out into the blood if you are losing bone mass. Because so much lead and aluminum is bound in the bones, lead and aluminum may not be accurately reflected in test results until the person ages and starts to lose bone mass. As people age and become osteopenic, there is an increased loss of bone. This causes a release of heavy metals that had been safely stored in their bones for decades.[259] You just have to keep repeating the chelation treatments. Eventually levels will drop when the bones have released all of the stored metals.

4. Increase alkalinity.

If you are too acid, your cells get sick, and you become more susceptible to disease. pH is an abbreviation for "potential hydrogen." pH is measured on a scale of 0-14, with 0 being the most acid and 14 being the most alkaline or basic. Alkaline water is the healthier water to drink. Get a pH test kit at the drug store. Tear off a strip and put it in your mouth first thing in the morning before eating or drinking anything. You can also test your pH two hours after a meal or drinking anything. If it turns green, you are alkaline. Yellow, orange, or red mean that your saliva is too acid. Ideally, your pH should be at least 6.5 or above at least once a day. If your test strip reads on the acid side, change your lifestyle to raise your pH.

To become more alkaline:

- Exercise.
- Don't drink acidic water--bottled water or any water that has fluoride and/or chlorine in it.
- Drink plenty of pure water.
- Don't drink soda pop, caffeinated, or alcoholic drinks.
- Grow wheatgrass, juice it, drink it, and do rectal implants (retain in colon).
- Eat as many raw vegetables and fruits as possible. Cut down on cooked foods.
- Avoid processed foods completely. This includes sugar, artificial sweeteners, and pasteurized milk.
- Avoid the bad fats (margarine, vegetable oil, canola oil, trans-fats, and hydrogenated oils).
- Eat plenty of the good fats (butter, olive oil, flax oil, avocados, nuts, and seeds).
- Take plenty of minerals. Include calcium, magnesium, zinc, and trace minerals.
- Baking soda baths (2 cups) are very alkalinizing.

5. Avoid EMR.

If you live in the city, you can find out if the electromagnetic fields around you are responsible for your poor sleep by going out of town for a while to a place that is so remote that cell phones don't work. If you sleep well there, you have a clue.

Some people have had success blocking the electromagnetic radiation by lining workspace, living space, and sleeping space with aluminum insulation. Aluminum siding and an aluminum roof are also useful. Others have reported that sleeping with a mylar space blanket between sheet and blanket helps their sleep quality considerably.
- Unplug all electrical devices in your bedroom.
- No cell phones or cordless phones in your bedroom.

6. Continue to detox for life.

Good results from detoxification programs can be seen within ten days when people start a good program of detoxification and continue to follow through with it. If you feel sick or bad when starting a detox program, that just means that you need it very badly. Slow down the detoxification, and do repeated cycles of it. The longer you stick with it, the better you will feel. Because of the toxic environment and the difficulty in getting toxins out, it is necessary to continue on for the rest of your life if you want to experience radiant health. When levels of toxicity are extreme, such as in some cases of Parkinson's, it is important to get treatment using the FIR sauna and lymph drainage techniques at least three times a week. Even though improvement may be seen within a week or two, if you want to recover your health, you must continue on with the detox program for the rest of your life.

This is what happens when you stick with it:
- People lose fat.
- People have improvement in their senses. Clarity of vision improves. Sense of taste sharpens.
- Some people report hair growth in bald spots.
- Flexibility improves. Mobility improves. Pain in muscles and joints decreases.
- Strength increases.

B. TREAT INFECTIOUS DISEASE.

AFTER FINDING OUT WHAT KIND OF INVASION YOU HAVE, your physician will tell you how to eliminate it. There are some exotic parasites in this world, especially if you travel far and wide. If you have a microbe which seems to be resistant to everything with which you and your primary-care physician have tried, consult an anti-aging physician for a comprehensive treatment plan.

Vitamins in pharmacologic doses (high dosages much greater than available in diet) are very effective as anti-inflammatory, antibacterial, antiviral, and anti-cancer agents. Vitamin C is the prototype and has been used intravenously for the effective treatment of some cancers.[260] Taking a gram or two of vitamin C several times a day may be helpful in fighting viruses or bacteria that you didn't know you had.[261] Ascorbic acid or magnesium ascorbate powders are cheap sources of Vitamin C. Mix into juice or water and drink. When you get diarrhea, you've maxed out on water-soluble Vitamin C and your intestines can't absorb any more. Ascorbyl palmitate and Lypo-Spheric™ Vitamin C are fat-soluble forms that allow you to take larger quantities if needed to squelch nasty infections. Even Vitamin C may have complications, so work with your physician.

The Gut:
The gut is critical in getting rid of hormone metabolites. Dysbiosis is an overgrowth of yeast and bacteria in the gut. Dysbiosis impairs Phase 3 digestion, the digestion with bile salts and subsequent reabsorption. If you have impaired Phase 3 digestion (gall bladder), you have impaired excretion of hormones. Women with fibroids, which are an indication of estrogen dominance, frequently have dysbiosis.

The Mouth:
Maintain good hygiene with brushing and flossing and by using the water-pic-type appliances. Treatment for gum infections includes using a water pic after eating, flossing, and swishing diluted hydrogen peroxide around in your mouth. Gum infections often clear up when gut infections are treated. Remove mercury amalgams. Localized gingivitis and periodontitis (inflammation of the gums and alveolar bone loss) may occur around a tooth with a silver amalgam.

The Skin:
Don't use any toxic chemicals on your skin. Choose natural alternatives that are made only with healthy ingredients. Get out in the sun for short periods of time each day. Sunlight kills pathological bacteria on your skin.[262]

The Sinuses:

If you have periodic sinus infections, structural therapy with osteopathic cranialsacral therapy may return health to the sinuses. Often sutures that have been impacted by trauma calcify. Then only NeuroCranial Restructuring (NCR) or balloon-assisted cranial manipulation will relieve the compression.

Remove the source of the irritation with clean air machines. Often removing dietary allergens will help a person to overcome allergy to pollen in the air. Eating wheat commonly exacerbates hay fever. Try eliminating it for a few weeks to see if your allergies improve. Dairy products also cause a lot of mucus production in some people.

Infection hides in the mucous in the sinuses, so drying the secretions in the sinuses with decongestants may lead to chronic infection that requires antibiotics. If you get drainage of the sinuses, the body will heal without an antibiotic. If you do not get drainage, the antibiotic cannot penetrate infected mucous. Nasal washes and a Nettie Pot may be very useful. You may use sterile saline or herbal treatments (like golden seal) in the wash. Menthol is an effective decongestant that does not have the toxic effects of pharmaceuticals. Menthol and other natural remedies soothe the mucous production without blocking it. Natural mucolytics like slippery elm are indicated to get the mucous flowing and out.

1. Boost immunity.

When our immune systems become compromised, we are setting the stage for inflammatory disorders, cancer, infection, and early death. Infectious disease and environmental insults challenge our immunity.

Using vaccines are not always the best approach. Immunizations undoubtedly save thousands of lives each year and have eradicated terrible diseases from the planet. But we still must question possible adverse side effects and health problems as a result of this manipulation of our immune systems. Immunizations may be the best choice for you and your children or may be required, so measure the risk/benefit ratio of each vaccine that you choose. *Don't over-immunize and heal the adverse effects of immunizing with immune modulators.*

Immune modulators to overcome challenges:

- Andrographis paniculata.
- Acanthopanax senticosa.
- Green tea.
- Turmeric.
- Grape seed extract.
- Aloe Vera.
- Vitamin C.
- Beta glucan.
- Ashwagandha.
- Echinacea purpurea.
- Goldenseal.
- Zinc.
- Golden thread.
- Coriolus versicolor.
- Immunoglobulins.
- Astragalus.
- Siberian Ginseng.
- Garlic.
- Spirulina.
- Amla.
- Homeopathics.

2. Treat bacterial infections.

Killing pathogens with antibiotics is often necessary to overcome illness, but antibiotics come with their own set of problems. Antibiotics are the primary cause of the loss of healthy GIT flora and the overgrowth of other organisms. We stay in balance as long as the "good" bacteria keep the "bad" bacteria from overgrowing. If this balance is lost, it may never be recovered. During courses of antibiotics, drug-resistant organisms overgrow.

Appropriate use of probiotics for both bacteria and yeast following the course of antibiotics will recreate a healthy balance.[263] Anti-aging physicians recognize that treatment of dysbiosis is necessary for good health. Most state-of-the-art testing labs test for dysbiosis as a part of their GI profiles. These state-of-the-art tests also test for sensitivities in order to discover what natural substances will decrease the overgrowth of the drug-resistant organisms, especially yeasts.

If your physician finds a specific bacterial infection, take the antibiotics as prescribed. Then follow up with probiotics to restore the normal gut flora. Avoid drinking tap water that has not been filtered, as the chlorine kills gut bacteria, including the good gut bacteria. Continue to eat cultured food products like cow's milk yogurt (if no milk allergy exists) or goat's milk yogurt. Make sure that the product contains live cultures. It is easy to make your own yogurt.

3. Treat viral infections.

The homeopathic caveat, "Terrain everything, microbe nothing," is a good strategy. Do everything that you can to make the terrain (your body) inhospitable to the virus. Alkalinization of the body is one way of doing that. Avoid taking in toxins, especially alcohol, sugar, and drugs. Every spoke of the medicine wheel is a possibility including oriental medicine, homeopathy, allopathic medicine, naturopathic medicine, structural medicine, Ayurvedic medicine, and spiritual and emotional health.

"Silver sol" is silver in solution and is more active than colloidal silver. Silver sol will kill viruses when it contacts them. Be careful with it, as it kills all of the bacteria that it contacts. As viruses and bacteria are killed off in great numbers, you may experience detox reactions. Titrate the dose to a tolerable level that doesn't cause you too much distress. Take it in small doses for short periods of time with breaks in between treatments. Use it sparingly and follow up rounds of silver sol with probiotics and yogurt.

Other strategies include intravenous vitamin C, and anti virals, both allopathic and herbal. There are many treatments for viral infections in alternative medicine—electromagnetic, ozone, many anti-viral herbs, high-dose supplements, and homeopathics.

For acute or chronic viral infections, many anti-aging physicians recommend 100,000 I.U. of vitamin D3, 100,000 I.U. of vitamin A, and 10 grams of vitamin C each day for a few days. Check with your physician before trying this to ensure that it is safe for you. Work with an alternative medical practioner to develop a comprehensive treatment plan.

4. Treat parasites.

Patients often have three to five different parasites or worms and are relatively well with minimal symptoms. The immune system beats them down, but not out, and they hide in some little scar or pocket until your resistance weakens and then they grow back. They produce some gas and mild intestinal discomfort and maybe loose stools for a few days. Until they are eradicated, they continue to drain your energy.

Treatment usually requires allopathic drugs, but often the cure rate is far below 100% using only the drug of choice. Parasites are rugged little buggers and will hide out to evade eradication. To approach a 100% cure rate, *pre-treat* with natural anti-parasitic combinations like "Paraguard" *before* using the allopathic drug.

Complete eradication of infection is the only satisfactory result. Otherwise the infection just grows back. If your test results indicate parasites, take the strong prescription medicine(s) for as long as is recommended by your physician. Herbal remedies do not often permanently cure.

5. Treat leaky gut.

Treating leaky gut is important if a person has multiple food allergies and high inflammation. The standard of care followed by traditional physicians is that there is no such thing as leaky gut disease. If your physician is unaware of leaky gut syndrome, positive test results from doing the mannitol/lactulose test[264] might convince him/her of the diagnosis and direct proper therapy.

To treat leaky gut or intestinal malabsorption use the "4 R" plan:

Remove mucosal irritants such as allergenic foods, alcohol, gluten (if sensitive), and non-steroidal anti-inflammatory agents.
* Elimination diet.
* Remove possible pathogens (bacteria, yeast, parasites).
* Reduce sugar, refined carbohydrates, saturated fat, and red meat (may induce bacterial enzyme activity).
* Restore proper transit time. Increase dietary fiber (especially insoluble) and water.

Replace agents for digestive support:
* Pancreatic or plant enzymes, bile salts, betaine HCl, digestive herbs, or disaccharidases.

Reinoculate with friendly bacteria if low:
* Probiotic supplementation, including Lactobacilli and Bifidobacteria.
* Fructooligosaccharides and inulin to enhance growth of friendly flora.

Repair mucosal lining:
* Glutamine and L-arginine are amino acids that help to regenerate gut linings. Also take EFAs, zinc, pantothenic acid, Vitamins C, E, beta carotene, N-acetyl glucosamine, gamma oryzanol, glycerrhiza, and aloe vera.
* Anti-inflammatories, like quercetin and pycnogenol, are recommended.
* Butyric acid is a short chain fatty acid made in the intestines when fiber is fermented by bacteria. Supplementation with butyric acid helps to repair damaged cells.
* Free radical scavengers are also helpful. They include Vitamin E, beta carotene, ascorbic acid, zinc, selenium, superoxide dismutase, carotenoids, glutathione, N-acetyl cysteine, pycnogenol, and flavonoids.
* Saccharomyces boulardii, whey globulin concentrate, or bovine colostrum to improve local immunity.
* Ginkgo biloba to enhance circulation to intestinal epithelium.
* Optimize overall nutrition.

6. Treat heartburn.

Heartburn may be caused by inadequate stomach acid OR excess stomach acid. If you suffer from heartburn, your physician must distinguish between deficient or excessive hydrochloric acid.

Inadequate stomach acid (hydrochloric acid) is impaired Phase I digestion and results in putrification in the intestines. This poor digestion results in heartburn. If you have deficient hydrochloric acid, which is usually found in older people without a history of hyperacidity, the use of betaine hydrochloride will resolve the poor digestion. B12 deficiency is often associated with deficient hydrochloric acid.

Excessive hydrochloric acid should be treated with antacids and proton pump inhibitors until the underlying cause can be corrected. Heartburn is most often related to dietary indiscretion, stress, and excessive alcohol consumption. Try eating small, frequent meals. Avoid irritating foods like spices. Sleep propped-up if you have reflux.

7. Treat yeast.

If your stool test indicates that you have a yeast overgrowth, you may be able to overcome the yeast by following the anti-candida diet and taking anti-yeast herbals. As yeast thrives on sugar and fermented foods, treatment always involves diet. This mainly involves removing all sugar (breads, fruit, etc.), white foods (flour, rice, potatoes), and fermented foods. Herbal remedies are very helpful and many are available. Often a natural anti-parasitic combination, like Paraguard, produces good yeast coverage. The probiotic for yeast overgrowth is Saccharomyces boulardii, and is often taken with MOS (mannan oligosaccharides), a prebiotic.

A variety of anti-yeast drugs are available including the big gun, Diflucan, (fluconazole). Intermediate treatment would be nystatin, a drug that kills yeast but is not absorbed by the intestine into the blood.

8. Treat dysbiosis.

After removing bacterial overgrowth, parasitic and fungal infections, and cleansing the GI tract with enemas, colonics, and colonic cleansing preparations such as psyllium and bentonite clay, it is time to establish a healthy microflora environment, so that food can be properly digested. When antibiotics are taken, the bacterial balance of the gut is thrown out of balance.

- *Normalize the flora with probiotics.* Re-colonize the intestines using probiotics. Probiotics reduce the formation of colon cancers[265] and bladder cancer. Take a probiotic before eating. Using a probiotic primes immune function, reduces yeast, and helps you to absorb nutrients in food.
- *Take prebiotics (FOSs) to support the healthy growth of the probiotics.* Using probiotics and prebiotics may be especially important in overcoming obesity.
- *Improve digestion with digestive enzymes if deficient.* Digestive enzymes break down food for absorption into the body. Use betaine hydrochloride and pepsin for deficient Phase I digestion (stomach) and pancreatic enzymes for deficient Phase II digestion (pancreas).
- *Reduce the intake of:*
  - o Animal proteins.
  - o High carbohydrate meals.
  - o Processed food.

C. TREAT HORMONAL DYSFUNCTION.

YOU WILL HAVE SICK METABOLISM UNTIL YOU BALANCE YOUR HORMONES. Treat insulin resistance, treat adrenal and thyroid dysfunctions, optimize sex hormones, correct the causes of faulty estrogen metabolism, optimize human growth hormone, and restore leptin and ghrelin sensitivity.

1. Treat insulin resistance.

Insulin resistance underlies the formation of toxic belly fat (TBF) and is created by toxic belly fat. Treat metabolic syndrome as early as possible, even before the full syndrome has manifested. The goal is to overcome insulin resistance and to become sensitive to insulin again. Treat it with hormone optimization, diet, lifestyle, supplementation, and possibly pharmacotherapy. Once the disease progresses to a late stage, treatment with diet, exercise, and nutrition are helpful, but the severity of the condition will also require the use of drugs. If you notice your waist size growing, begin to change your lifestyle immediately.

In early type II diabetes, the predominant problem is pathologic cellular metabolism caused by insulin resistance and toxicity. Early type II diabetes can be reversed. In insulin-resistant people, the high insulin levels push the pancreas into burnout. *If the pancreas becomes burned out, then type II diabetes is irreversible and becomes type I diabetes, requiring insulin injections.*

Treatment for all stages of dysglycemia (impaired sugar):
- Optimize hormones.
- Increase physical activity.[266]
- Diet--low glycemic, high fiber, omega-3s, monounsaturated fatty acids (MUFAs) as in olive oil and avocados, antioxidants, fish, vegetables, nuts, seeds.
- Lose weight.
- Manage stress (relaxation, biofeedback, slow rhythmic breathing, and meditation).
- Get plenty of sleep.
- Remove toxicity.
- Identify and address all causes of inflammation.

Increase physical activity.

The mainstay of treatment begins with exercise. You can do everything else, but if you do not exercise, you cannot become insulin-sensitive again (fasting blood sugar less than 90). If this is very difficult for you, or if you have serious health issues that impair your ability to exercise, be supervised by your physician and begin with cardiac rehabilitation.

If you can walk fifteen minutes, start with that and add one minute a week. But you must DO IT EVERY DAY, WITHOUT FAIL. We all have fifteen minutes a day. If you get out of the door, and you just can't do it that day, that counts as a successful day. If you get out and feel better and feel like walking thirty minutes, that is even better. But never miss a day. If you cannot walk, see your physician and physical therapist for a program and exercise in water, if available. Ninety minutes of moderate-intensity exercise (walking briskly) within two hours of a meal has been shown to lower triglycerides and glucose levels by 50%. Exercise aerobically at least thirty minutes daily. Gradually add in thirty minutes of weight training three times per week with core exercises to reduce belly fat.

Diet.

Balancing carbohydrates with protein and fat is the key to weight normalization and insulin sensitivity. Advice to always eat carbohydrate buffered with fat and protein is well-founded in physiology. When fat and protein accompany carbohydrates, the glycemic load (sugar) is slowed and satiety is established. In order to produce the satiety hormones that counter increased insulin and to achieve a low ratio of insulin to glucagon, buffer all carbohydrates with protein and fat. Keep carbohydrate portions small (15 grams if you are insulin-resistant).

Keeping a low ratio of insulin to glucagon is an important strategy to follow to heal sick metabolism. To lose weight and reverse metabolic syndrome, we need to lower insulin and raise glucagon. Insulin is a most powerful growth factor and is the hormone of energy storage. Glucagon is the hormone of energy utilization and release. Insulin moves glucose into storage (glycogen in the liver and fat in the adipocyte). A meal high in carbohydrate produces an insulin/glucagon ratio of 70 where a meal low in carbohydrate produces a ratio of 7.

The hormones of satiety are produced only by fat and protein intake. Two hormones not only produce satiety, but also stimulate glucagon secretion: gastrin and CCK. Gastrin is a hormone produced in significant amounts in the stomach and stimulates gastric secretions and emptying. It stimulates glucagon production when protein is eaten but not carbohydrate. CCK (cholecystokinin) is secreted by the GI tract in response to protein and fat and promotes gall bladder contractions, pancreatic enzymes, and increased motility. It also increases glucagon secretion (a good thing).

Peptide YY has food intake-inhibiting activity and is released by fat intake. Secretin, stimulated by protein intake, increases pancreatic secretion and inhibits glucagon secretion. Neurotensin is released by fat intake and inhibits intestinal motility.

The hormones produced from carbohydrate intake are the potent stimulators of insulin secretion and make you fat. Insulin's job is to store the sugar. This makes you fatter.

The most important stimulators of insulin secretion are the hormones GIP and GLP-1, which are produced when carbohydrate is eaten. GIP is gastric inhibitory peptide and it slows the stomach down in response to glucose and fat. GLP-1 (glucagon-like polypeptide-1) is the insulin stimulator of the beta islet cells of the pancreas and, with GIP, is the most important GI tract stimulator of insulin.

Control, but do not completely eliminate carbs. The goals are to restore a healthy insulin to glucagon ratio and put the body in a glucagon mode (energy expenditure), not an insulin mode (energy storage).

Eat a snack or small meal every 4 hours. Always include a small amount of carbohydrate. If you are insulin-resistant, eat 15 grams of carbohydrate, not more or less, with protein and good fats. A 15-gram carbohydrate feeding is one slice of bread, or a small apple.

Always eat low-glycemic carbs. The diet should focus on protein and vegetables, and keeping carbohydrates and glycemic index low. Increase soluble fiber intake and healthy fats. Avoid soft drinks, trans fats, sugar, refined carbohydrates, and fructose, especially high-fructose corn syrup. Only drink fruit juices and milk very sparingly, if at all. Take omega 3s and mono-unsaturated fatty acids (MUFAs), as in avocados, antioxidants, fish, vegetables, nuts, and seeds.

Foods that will decrease glucose and insulin:

- **Onions** lower glucose by competing with insulin, increasing insulin activity.
- **Brewer's yeast** is high in chromium which helps insulin bind to the cell receptors.
- **Cinnamon** may act as an insulin substitute and reduces blood sugar 20 to 30 percent.
- **Olive oil** improves blood sugar control while lowering triglycerides.
- **Beans, legumes, and nuts** have fiber which improves glucose tolerance and insulin sensitivity.
- **Mangoes** have a low glycemic index, high fiber, and high enzymes.

Gain blood sugar control with diet and supplements. Chromium is especially important for insulin sensitivity, and most overweight people test low for it. **High-dose alpha lipoic acid,** the universal antioxidant, is effective for diabetic neuropathy. See your physician for appropriate testing and supplement recommendations.

Make sure that you are getting plenty of vitamins, phytonutrients, minerals, and trace minerals to build hormones and run good metabolism. Co-factors may come from berries, greens, fruits, and vegetables. Phytonutrients are powerful antioxidants that enhance immune response, cause apoptosis (destruction) of cancer cells, repair DNA damage caused by toxins, and detoxify carcinogens.

Vitamin requirements will be much higher for those who engage in strenuous exercise, smokers, substance abusers, prescription-drug users, diabetics, and those with chronic inflammation. *Trace minerals* have been depleted from the soil. Therefore it is increasingly difficult to get the trace minerals you need just from eating food anymore. The most important trace minerals are chromium, boron, vanadium, zinc, and selenium. Take B vitamins, vitamin D, biotin, magnesium, zinc, chromium, vanadium, alpha-lipoic acid, antioxidants, fish oils, green tea, cinnamon, maitake, citrus bergamot, gymnema, oat beta glucans, corosolic acid, fenugreek, and DHEA if needed.

2. Treat adrenal dysfunction.

People with stage 2-3 adrenal fatigue may have normal or low morning salivary cortisol levels. But their noon and 5 pm cortisol levels are at the bottom of the normal range or below. If the hormones that they're using to make cortisol (DHEA) are all low, this will result in lower testosterone and estrogen. This is indicative of stage 3 adrenal fatigue. Lack of a cortisol peak at 8 am suggests hypothalamic/pituitary dysfunction.

Treatment methods for adrenal dysfunction include:
- **Stress reduction techniques. Lifestyle--stop over-working, dieting, over-exercising, taking caffeine, drugs.**
- **Sleep hygiene--only use your bed for sleep and sex.**
- **Plant adaptogens and herbal supplements.**
- **Vitamins and minerals.**
- **Glandular extracts.**
- **Pharmacologic therapy—physiologic doses of hydrocortisol (Cortef) for stage 4 dysfunction.**

Stress reduction techniques. First identify and eliminate your stressors. Change your attitude or response to the stressor. Don't let it get to you. Reframe your outlook. Have an attitude of gratitude. Eat regular meals and chew your food carefully. Do gentle exercise like Tai Chi, Yoga, and Pilates. Develop a spiritual or religious practice. Modify your diet to decrease inflammation (especially decrease omega-6 oils—vegetable oils). Eat protein and at least 15 grams of carbohydrate four to six times a day. Meditate. Take frequent breaks from your work. Stop time-urgent behavior.

Sleep hygiene. Insomnia is common. Support sleep.
- If exercise ramps you up, don't exercise at night. Exercise regularly, but don't over exercise.
- Don't do anything in your bed except for sex or sleep.
- Don't do stimulating things three hours before bed.
- Put on quiet music and turn lights down about an hour before bed.
- Before bed, take lecithin, glycine, and phosphatidylserine to combat high nighttime cortisol.
- Take melatonin to help with sleep.
- Don't watch TV or stay on the computer when it is bedtime.
- Go to sleep early.

Adaptogens promote resistance to stress, fatigue, trauma, and anxiety. They normalize cortisol levels, maintain homeostasis, and enhance immune function. They protect end organs, like heart and brain, from chronic stress hormone elevation. In order of effectiveness:
- **Ashwagandha** is the premier adaptogen. It protects heart and brain, reduces tumor cell proliferation, and scavenges free radicals. Take it in the afternoon or night as powder, tincture, tea, capsule, or tablet.
- **Rhodiola rosea** is an antidepressant, decreases pain, improves mental function, the immune system, endurance, adrenal and cardiovascular function, and heals gut inflammation.
- **Relora** is a proprietary blend.
- **Panax ginseng** is energizing. 4-7% is a good quality extract of ginsenosides.
- **Siberian ginseng or eleutherococcus senticosus** may be energizing. It gives endurance, is an immunostimulant, an antidepressant, stimulates ACTH production, and prevents oxidative stress. It normalizes blood pressure and cortisol. It improves cholesterol, focus,

concentration, and reaction time. It suppresses inflammation and DNA damage. It is stimulating, so don't take it too late in the day.

- **Magnolia officinalis** relaxes, improves mood, and reduces stress.
- **Holy Basil leaf** stimulates insulin secretion, protects the pancreas, is an antioxidant, free radical scavenger, and protects your heart during stress. Take it in the evening.
- **Glycyrrhiza** protects mitochondria (where cells make energy) during oxidative stress.
- **Maca** improves sperm production and motility and improves homeostasis.
- **Astragalus** helps glucose, the immune system, and heals gut inflammation.
- **Cordyceps** is mildly sedative. Take daily.
- **Phellodendron amurense** is an anti-inflammatory Chinese adaptogen.
- **Schizandra berry** is mildly energizing, improves libido, helps the lungs, helps detox the liver, increases endurance, mental function, reduces fatigue, helps with mood, infectious diseases, hypotension, allergic dermatitis, and G.I. diseases.

Herbal Supplements:
- **Theanine** is a calming amino acid that optimizes dopamine, GABA, and serotonin to deal with stress. The more you take, the more your alpha waves increase. Green tea contains 1-3% Theanine. It decreases norepinephrine, lowering blood pressure.
- **Phosphatidylserine** lowers high night-time cortisol levels when taken at bedtime. Phosphatidylserine is a phospholipid that is a component of cell membranes. It improves mood, lowers cortisol from physical stress, and prevents stress-induced memory loss.

Vitamins and minerals for the adrenals include:
- **Vitamin C** reduces high cortisol and blood pressure.
- **Pantothine** is activated pantothenic acid, vitamin B-5.
- **Magnesium** glycinate or citrate. Magnesium is involved in over 300 enzymatic pathways, and reduces ACTH secretion at night.
- **L-tyrosine** is the precursor for dopamine, epinephrine, and norepinephrine. **N-Acetyl Tyrosine** is a more bioavailable form of L-tyrosine.
- **Methionine and s-adenosylmethionine** (SAMe) help to make epinephrine.

 Glandular extracts may help the adrenals and other aging endocrine glands to recover. Taken in excessive dosages, they will decrease your own production of hormones. Don't use them instead of seeking medical treatment.

 Pharmacologic therapy. Cortef is bioidentical cortisol.[267] Physiologic cortisol supplementation only gives the body the minimal steroid support that the adrenals cannot provide in stage 4 adrenal exhaustion. It puts the adrenals at rest and improves the health of all systems. But to *heal* the adrenals, a full treatment plan is required. Without making the lifestyle changes, anything else will be minimally effective. Low-dose Cortef rests the adrenal glands and supports the body while lifestyle changes, adaptogens, and other treatment methods *heal* the adrenals. It improves cellular immunity. Taking physiologic doses of natural cortisol, (Cortef) in divided doses will not suppress the adrenal glands or cause any side effects. It may take eight months to a year or sometimes longer to heal your adrenals. After eight months to a year, keep using the vitamins and herbs to heal the adrenals, but your doctor will taper off the natural cortisol.

 If the pituitary is the source for the stage 4 adrenal dysfunction, it may not be possible to discontinue the Cortef. If you haven't healed and responded to the treatment, there is something that hasn't been addressed, like heavy metals, receptor resistance, adaptive or protective hypocortisolism, or nutritional deficiencies. If you don't make lifestyle changes, treatment of adrenal dysfunction will not be successful.

 If DHEA tests come back low, it may indicate that DHEA is being used to make cortisol. Supplementation with DHEA would be indicated while treating the adrenal dysfunction.

Adrenal Stress--Stage 1-3 Treatment Plan:

- Cortisol is too high. You cannot treat adrenal dysfunction without making lifestyle changes. Address lifestyle by eliminating stress and adding meditation. Do things to calm down. Stop worrying. Stop being angry.
- If morning cortisol is too high, take phosphatidylserine in the a.m. If morning *and* night cortisol levels are too high, take phosphatidylserine morning and evening.
- Pace your activities to allow time between commitments. Avoid time urgency. Get help with coping skills, overcoming coping liabilities, and setting limits on time. See a counselor or therapist who knows stress reduction techniques.
- Stop drinking coffee and avoid stimulants.
- Eat every four hours. Avoid high-protein, no or low carbohydrate diets.
- Adaptogens bring cortisol into the normal range, heal the injured adrenals, and protect organs injured by stress, especially the brain and heart. Use adaptogens without Cortef. If really tired and not anxious, use a neutral or stimulating adaptogen.
- Replace DHEA and pregnenolone as needed and balance sex hormones.
- Use detox protocols.
- Curtail alcohol use. Introduce calming herbs to replace alcohol use.
- Exercise.

Adrenal Exhaustion--Stage 4 Treatment Plan:

- This stage is characterized by low cortisol and depleted reserves of upstream and downstream hormones. A trial of Cortef may be both diagnostic and therapeutic.
- Use adrenal glandulars or Cortef along with adaptogens, unless protective adrenal dysfunction exists, or there is receptor resistance with dumping of cortisol.
- Use full range of adaptogens and a low glycemic diet.
- Restrict exercise.
- Replace the neurotransmitter precursors that are depleted, especially tryptophan.
- Assure adequate sleep. Rest is essential.
- Minimize stress of all types—all ability to respond to stress is gone.

3. Treat thyroid dysfunction.

The epidemic of hypothyroidism is largely being caused by chronic stress, poor lifestyle, and environmental toxicity.[268] The diagnosis of hypothyroidism is also becoming more common because previously it was underdiagnosed. Clinical symptoms are more important than TSH (thyroid stimulating hormone) levels and thyroid blood test numbers.

Treat and support the adrenals first. The thyroid is responsible for making energy in the cells. Apparent thyroid problems often clear up when treating the adrenals. An imbalance of cortisol may mask itself as a thyroid problem.

Treat estrogen dominance as well as the thyroid. High estrogen levels in perimenopause are often associated with thyroid problems. Thyroid function may improve when estrogen dominance is corrected by increasing progesterone. Treating estrogen dominance with soy is not optimal because soy may worsen hypothyroidism and only treats the symptoms of estrogen dominance, not the cause.

High levels of estrogen cause an increase in thyroid-binding globulin (TBG) which causes symptoms of low thyroid—cold, sluggish, tired. Even if thyroid tests are normal, some physicians may prescribe thyroid meds. These patients still don't feel better, because the estrogen dominance that is causing the thyroid problem has not been treated.

You can't make thyroid hormone without iodine. Most Americans are terribly deficient in iodine, as they don't get enough in their diets. The average amount of iodine in the Japanese diet is 12.5 milligrams (mg) a day. Iodized salt provides only about 400 micrograms (mcg) per teaspoon. You can get iodine by eating seafood and iodine supplements. *Taking iodine daily will help to metabolize excess estrogen, reduce breast tenderness caused by estrogen dominance, and clear halogen (chlorine, bromine, fluoride) toxicity.*

4. Bioidentical Hormone Replacement Therapy (BHRT).

You can choose to be healthy, active, and vibrant right up to the very end of your life if you replace your missing hormones with bioidentical ones, eat right, and exercise.

- BHRT keeps the endocrine system healthy, which is essential to vitality and well-being.
- BHRT may restore libido and vitality, leading to a better, closer relationship. BHRT can preserve a happy marriage, allowing both partners to live life to its fullest.
- BHRT diminishes heart disease, strokes, and osteoporosis. Heart disease kills 31% of all American white women ages 50-94. *Heart attacks and strokes each kill more women than breast cancer and endometrial cancer combined.*
- Bioidentical hormones are relatively safe because they are identical to the hormones made in our own bodies. We can take precautions to keep our cancer risk low, an option that is not available with synthetic and horse hormones.

5. Women: replace sex hormones.

Menopausal and perimenopausal women who choose to use bioidentical sex hormones to simulate the hormones of a young, cycling, reproductive woman have reported great benefits in health, mood, sexual interest, and weight normalization.[269] [270] Do not use "hormone" products that are sold on the internet. Bioidentical hormones are only available by prescription. Do it right. Don't mess around with something as important as your hormones.

Find a doctor who specializes in BHRT

If your test results indicate that your estrogen and progesterone levels are inadequate, begin BHRT. Begin BHRT at first signs of deficiency to avoid the hormonal imbalances of the perimenopausal state, which is a dangerous time for women (estrogen dominance with increased prolactin and insulin). Testosterone may be needed, so be sure to test for it. Your anti-aging doctor will replace it if levels are low.

A physician who is knowledgeable in bioidentical hormone balancing is needed to manage the balance of estrogen, progesterone, and testosterone. It is important to find a physician who really understands women's hormones, knows when and how to check hormone levels, and is not afraid to prescribe BHRT.

Bioidentical hormone replacement is not taught in medical school, nor is it standard of care for *women.* Many physicians do not understand the difference between bioidentical hormones, which are hormones that have the exact shape as those manufactured in our own bodies, and horse and synthetic hormones, which are seen as foreign by our bodies. These physicians use the term, "estrogen," when they prescribe "Premarin," a horse estrogen from <u>pregnant mare's urine</u>. They use the term, "progesterone" to refer to various synthetic variants which include progestins, progestogens, and gestagens. Progestins and progesterone are used as synonyms in many studies and books written by MDs. *"Provera" is not progesterone,* but a synthetic hormone. There are many other synthetic forms of estrogen and synthetic variants of progesterone and combinations of them. Traditional physicians call them *all* HRT or Hormone Replacement Therapy. Nothing could be further from the truth (unless you are a horse). Humans cannot "replace" their lost hormones with horse hormones or synthetic hormones which our bodies do not recognize.

Since most of the studies that have been done on HRT have studied women taking horse and synthetic hormones, traditional doctors are leery of using bioidentical hormones because they don't understand the difference. The verbiage in the studies using pharmaceutically-manufactured progestins often erroneously refers to these progestins as "progesterone."

Doctors reading these studies conclude that progesterone is responsible for multiple health risks, when it was actually the use of synthetic progestins that caused the problems.

Synthetic and horse hormones should not be used. Because *their shapes are foreign to our bodies,* our enzyme systems cannot prevent their damaging effects at the receptor site. The human body cannot efficiently excrete them. *Premarin is not safe* because the human body metabolizes the horse estrogen as a foreign substance into dangerous metabolites. Women who use synthetic hormones like Prempro are at a much greater risk for breast cancer and heart attacks. They throw the body out of balance and lead to illness.

Estrogen replacement.

When estrogen is deficient in women, supplementing with estradiol helps bones and teeth and increases serotonin levels, improving mood. It maintains collagen in the skin, decreases itchy skin, dry hair, wrinkles, and tooth loss. It increases the metabolism, insulin sensitivity, and muscle mass. The use of transdermal, bioidentical estradiol prevents the negative metabolic shifts that are associated with menopause. It prevents brain deterioration, improves blood flow, reduces blood pressure, lowers homocysteine,[271] and decreases incidence of heart attack and stroke. It slows the formation of perioral wrinkles. It has a huge effect on mood and thinking, decreasing risk of Alzheimer's. It improves concentration, helps with fine motor skills, and increases sexual interest.

Progesterone replacement.

Supplementation with natural bioidentical progesterone restores hormonal balance, especially during estrogen dominance. The two hormones, estrogen and progesterone, rise and fall throughout the menstrual cycle. Keeping them balanced is important for a woman's health, well-being, and state of mind. When there is not enough progesterone in relation to estrogen, a woman develops estrogen dominance, which causes many health problems.

Females who are menopausal are usually estrogen-deficient and estrogen-dominant. This means they have low estrogen levels and need more, but have even lower progesterone. To raise estrogen and make them more estrogen-dominant without raising progesterone can be a dangerous thing to do. Estrogen dominance is associated with endometrial cancer and raises the risk of breast cancer.

Replacing progesterone when it is low in states of perimenopause or menopause will reduce inflammation and chronic degenerative diseases. While estrogen levels drop only 40-60% at menopause, progesterone levels may drop to near zero in some women. *It is best given only during days 14-28 of the menstrual cycle, to simulate normal cycles.* Bioidentical progesterone can only be obtained *by prescription.*

Don't replace estrogen without replacing progesterone as well. Estrogen is proliferative, which means it builds things. In the body, tissues that are built up have to be taken down again or they will cause trouble. This is where progesterone comes in. Progesterone removes the garbage. If estrogen is given without progesterone, it is called "unopposed estrogen" and may lead to cancer. If your doctor wants to give you estrogen cream for vaginal dryness without giving you progesterone, this is not OK. It will lead to estrogen dominance or make it worse if you have it, which most women of all ages do.

Treat estrogen dominance.

For estrogen dominance in women, the hormonal intervention is bioidentical progesterone. *A diet high in soy and phytoestrogens may decrease symptoms of estrogen dominance, but does nothing to heal the disorder.* Take fiber with the highest-fat meal of the day to eliminate excess estrogen and toxicity. Adding two to four grams of fish or krill oil per day to the diet is helpful to lower inflammation.

Calcium D-glucarate helps to correct estrogen excess[272] caused by xenoestrogens. Because of all the xenoestrogens coming in from environmental pollutants like plastic, cosmetics, insecticides, and pesticides, most people have a huge toxic load of chemical hormones circulating in the body, and there's no way for the body to get rid of them.

Calcium D-glucarate helps both women and men to eliminate a lot of these xenoestrogens, carcinogens, and tumor promoters. Women who are trying to get pregnant may get pregnant after using it for a few months. It gets rid of excess estrogen quickly. Make sure to use enough. Be careful, it *may* interfere with some prescription antidepressants.

Oral estrogens should not be used.

Even if they are bioidentical, oral estrogens have undesirable effects. They are removed 60-80% by first-pass through the liver and metabolized into cancer-promoting chemicals. So you have to use three to four times more estrogen orally compared to sublingual or transdermal preparations. Oral estrogens increase body fat, triglycerides, raise blood pressure, insulin resistance, blood clots, gallbladder disease, C-reactive protein (an inflammatory marker), and increase cancer risk. Transdermal (creams, patch, or gels) estrogens are easy to use. Transdermal estrogens decrease fat, triglycerides, insulin resistance, and vascular resistance without increasing C-reactive protein.[273]

Testosterone?

Adding testosterone may be helpful but may make problems worse if it isn't really needed. In both men and women who have estrogen dominance, adding additional testosterone will increase the estrogen dominance because some of the increased testosterone will convert into estrogen, especially with belly fat. Estrogen dominance may look the same as low testosterone. *Doctors may confuse estrogen dominance with low androgens. It is important to measure estrogen, progesterone, and testosterone levels before supplementing with testosterone.*

Women who have low levels of testosterone may benefit from testosterone replacement. Your physician can give you a prescription that may be filled at a compounding pharmacy. The compounding pharmacy will make a cream in a strength to match your individual requirements using testosterone and/or DHEA that is rubbed into the skin once a day.

Maca is an herb used to boost testosterone levels. The effects of this Peruvian "ginseng" may be quite dramatic. It increases muscle mass, strength, and increases bone mineral density.[274]

6. Treat andropause.

Males who are truly hypogonadal (testosterone below the reference range) need hormone replacement therapy (HRT). Depression, decreased strength, inability to lose weight, and self-defeating behavior are symptoms of deficient testosterone. Start with HRT, and then lifestyle changes will be made much more successfully. Suboptimal testosterone levels may respond to lifestyle change, exercise, diet, weight loss, and altering self-defeating behavior. This may be all that is necessary to optimize testosterone levels. If lifestyle changes are not adequate, work with your anti-aging physician to add in HRT to optimize testosterone. If estrogen levels are still increased after diet and lifestyle changes, use an aromatase inhibitor (anastrozole). If 16-hydroxy metabolites are increased, use DIM.

Manipulating the hormone levels of an older man to match those of a young man may help his health considerably. Certainly the studies show that longevity increases as testosterone increases. We don't know what the average testosterone levels of a 60-year-old man were 1000 years ago or even 150 years ago. But they were probably not as low as the levels of today's average 60-year-old man. Our toxic environment and sedentary lifestyle may be responsible for this testosterone level drop.

Sexual dysfunction may be caused by heart meds. Cardiovascular disease, its complications, and its treatment are the biggest cause of sexual dysfunction. Find out if the meds you are taking are affecting your sexual performance and start a cardiac rehab program.

Seek therapy if necessary. Depression may be disguised as chronic anger, irritability, and hostility. Job loss, demotion, and approach of retirement may be depressing. If you must take antidepressants, find out if they will affect sexual performance. Seek natural alternatives first.

Causes of low androgen (male hormone) states include:

- Adrenal dysfunction with low DHEA.
- High estrogen levels produce a relatively-low androgen state.
- Insulin resistance.
- Sleep apnea.
- High Sex Hormone Binding Globulin (SHBG).
- Suppression of the hypothalamic-pituitary axis produces hypogonadotropic hypogonadism. Pituitary stimulation of the testes is inadequate. Treatment includes hCG (human chorionic gonadotropin) or testosterone. HCG acts like LH (luteinizing hormone), the hormone that is secreted by the pituitary to stimulate testosterone production from the testes. Using hCG is relatively safe for men and avoids the possible adverse effects of testosterone replacement therapy (see below).
- Reduced testicular response to LH with aging. This is hypergonadotropic hypogonadism. The testes are being stimulated to produce testosterone, but can't respond. Treatment is testosterone replacement therapy.

Testosterone replacement therapy.

Testosterone protects men against cancer. Uninformed men resist getting testosterone replacement therapy for fear of *getting* cancer. Uniformed doctors are reluctant to treat with testosterone if prostate problems are present. Testosterone replacement therapy does not cause prostate cancer.[275][276][277]

Testosterone replacement therapy doesn't hurt the prostate.[278] (Increased *estrogen* may produce prostatic symptoms.) Increased DHT is associated with prostatic hypertrophy (swollen prostate). If prostatic hypertrophy is present, blocking the conversion of testosterone to DHT will protect the prostate (see DHT section below).

When testosterone drops below levels needed to maintain health, testosterone replacement can work miracles in making a man younger, more productive, and more virile again. Andropausal men who use supplemental testosterone to bring their levels up to normal levels for a twenty or thirty-year-old experience great health benefits, greatly improved sexual function,[279] and improvement in chronic illnesses. Inflammatory conditions like arthritis, colitis, asthma, and heart disease decrease.

Testosterone replacement for hypogonadal men is safe and extremely beneficial.

- Testosterone decreases inflammation and lowers total cholesterol.[280]
- Testosterone improves cardiac function.[281][282][283] It improves symptoms of coronary artery disease.[284][285] Testosterone improves stamina and cardiac pump function.
- Testosterone may normalize blood pressure.[286]
- Testosterone improves glucose and body composition--more muscle, less fat.[287][288]
- Testosterone improves mood. Testosterone works even when antidepressants don't.[289]
- Testosterone reverses osteoporosis. It may improve osteoarthritis and rheumatoid arthritis.
- Testosterone improves cognitive function.[290][291] It improves blood flow in the brain.[292] It may prevent Alzheimer's disease.[293] Alzheimer's patients improve with testosterone.[294]
- Testosterone restores sex drive, orgasm, nocturnal erections, and libido.[295] It improves and may resolve erectile dysfunction.[296][297]
- Testosterone increases GH secretion by 10-20%.[298]

When taking testosterone replacement, don't go too high with testosterone or you'll feel great for a month and then crash because it may downregulate the testosterone receptors. Putting progesterone into the testosterone base may make men feel better because the progesterone blocks estrogen. It also reduces stress levels.

Decrease aromatization.

Giving testosterone replacement therapy without decreasing aromatase activity will raise estrogen and decrease the overall balance of male hormones. When testosterone is given to men who have abdominal fat, their abdominal fat may increase, because enzymes (aromatases) in that abdominal fat may turn testosterone into estrogen, which causes more abdominal fat. In andropause, aromatase produced by toxic belly fat turns what little testosterone a man has left into estrogen. This causes estrogen dominance in men. Too much estrogen in relationship to testosterone in men is dangerous. It leads to increased risk of prostate cancer. 16-hydroxylation of estrogen from bad estrogen metabolism produces a very significant risk of prostate cancer.

It may be best to treat the elevated level of estrogen and DHT by lowering the dose of testosterone. Excessive doses of testosterone may induce testosterone receptor resistance. In this instance, increased testosterone not only *doesn't* improve symptoms of hypogonadism, but produces increased receptor resistance and *decreases* the effectiveness of testosterone (downregulates it).[299] [300]

Until the belly fat is lost in males, a small dose of an aromatase inhibitor is necessary to counter the elevated estrogen and its negative effects on male metabolism. There are natural aromatase inhibitors like chrysin, genistein, resveratrol, oleuropein, quercetin, naringenin, and apigenin, *but the most effective treatment is to see your doctor and get anastrazole.* Be careful not to block the production of estradiol to the point where it goes to zero. Men need some estrogen for bone, brain, cardiovascular health, and libido. Increases in estrogen primarily need to be treated if there are symptoms like prostate inflammation. Selective estrogen receptor modulators (like tamoxifen) are not a good choice because they suppress HGH and totally block estrogen receptors.[301]

Block DHT formation.

To increase testosterone levels and effectiveness and decrease masculinizing side effects, including prostatic hypertrophy and hair loss, block the conversion of testosterone to DHT. The formation of DHT may be slowed by taking drugs or supplements that bind 5-alpha reductase, an enzyme that converts testosterone into DHT. The drugs, finasteride and dutasteride inhibit 5-alpha reductase. But try supplements first, as they are quite effective. Supplements that inhibit 5-alpha reductase include: saw palmetto, green tea, polygonum multiflorum, zinc, and reishi mushrooms. Medium chain fatty acids such as those found in coconut and the kernel of many palm fruits have also been found to inhibit 5-alpha reductase.

7. Correct faulty estrogen metabolism.

Both men and women should correct faulty estrogen metabolism to lower their risks of reproductive organ cancer. We can change our chances of getting cancers by modifying estrogen metabolism, diet, and lifestyle. We need to encourage estrogen to be metabolized down the good estrogen metabolism pathway (2-hydroxylation)[302] [303] and then to be methylated so that the metabolites will be excreted and will not lead to cancer. When you change your estrogen pathways and increase methylation ability, you are lowering your cancer risk.[304] If the results from your estrogen metabolism test show that estrogen is being metabolized primarily down a bad (4-hydroxylation) or ugly (16-alpha-hydroxylation) pathway, take nutrients that help to change the pathway to the good one to protect yourself from breast cancer, prostate cancer, and other cancers.[305] DIM helps estrogen to be metabolized in a good way, preventing the development of certain cancers.[306]

8. Optimize Human Growth Hormone.

Adult human growth hormone deficiency (AGHD) is very rare. The low growth hormone values of AGHD are caused by pituitary/hypothalamic dysfunction.

Most older patients have suboptimal values. This is not the same as AGHD. Optimal values for a given person or age are subject to different interpretations. Most anti-aging physicians would consider the growth hormone levels of a thirty-year old as optimal targets for treating the older patient. The goals of treating older patients with suboptimal levels of growth hormone are to build muscle mass and bone mass, improve vitality, and heal degenerative disease. Physical findings are important when considering whether or not to treat suboptimal growth hormone levels. Osteopenia in a male with adequate to optimal testosterone levels would be one indication to optimize growth hormone.

Risk to benefit ratio is critical in the assessment of whether GH should be optimized and what form to use. Expense is also a factor, because cost varies greatly among different forms of GH replacement. The major consideration before using GH for each person is the risk of stimulating an occult neoplastic lesion to grow. Always remember that the use of GH involves the serious risk of cancer, and this risk should not be undertaken lightly. Once the risk assessment is made, choose the form of GH stimulation that is the safest. The secretagogues that stimulate your own GH production are safer than injected HGH or IGF-1.

9. Restore leptin sensitivity.

To restore leptin sensitivity:

- Lose weight.
- Begin an exercise program and control your diet by balancing all carbohydrates with protein, eating only small amounts of carbohydrates, eating plenty of good fats, and eating low-glycemic foods.
- Get plenty of sleep.
- Stress reduction will help, because stress raises cortisol. Continuously-high cortisol levels inhibit proper leptin functioning. Follow the adrenal treatment protocols.
- If Growth Hormone is low, it will affect leptin sensitivity. When GH levels are in the reference range for a young person, other hormones will work optimally.

10. Restore ghrelin sensitivity.

To restore ghrelin sensitivity:

- Lose weight.
- Stop eating anything with sugar in it--cane sugar, fructose, corn syrup--any kind of sugar.
- Eliminate processed flours, potatoes, and corn products.
- Eat small meals that have plenty of protein.

D. TREAT INFLAMMATION.

*B*ELLY FAT PRODUCES INFLAMMATION *by secreting inflammatory cytokines.* TNF-alpha and IL-6 are the major inflammatory cytokines from belly fat. Their effects are variable but broad spectrum and highly destructive.

The use of systemic enzyme therapy is helpful in many chronic inflammatory conditions. Systemic enzyme therapy is totally safe, so asking your physician about this would be appropriate. *Systemic enzymes are specific digestive enzymes* taken on an empty stomach (rutoside, trypsin, and bromelain). They remove inflammatory cytokines and immune complexes (garbage from inflammatory reactions) from the body.

Systemic enzyme therapy reduces inflammation. Systemic enzyme therapy typically begins to decrease inflammatory symptoms after three months. After nine months, inflammatory symptoms may resolve with no medications. Even in the absence of C-Reactive

Protein (CRP) elevation, systemic enzyme therapy may still be helpful, as many inflammatory processes do not elevate CRP.

Homeopathic therapy: Traumeel stimulates the formation of the body's own anti-inflammatory agents, including transformation growth factor-beta. Zeel effectively decreases chronic inflammation, but may take four to six weeks to provide significant pain relief.

Avoid allopathic anti-inflammatory drugs, because they block all of the prostaglandin systems in the body. This is harmful. Also healing is inflammation, and we don't want to block that.

AA/EPA ratio: Inflammatory cytokines are built from fatty acids, and the average American diet is excessively high in pro-inflammatory fats. Omega-6 oils (vegetable oils) are proinflammatory and Omega-3 oils form the anti-inflammatory cytokines. Measurement of the AA/EPA ratio is a common measurement of proinflammatory status.

Treat Inflammation:

- Follow dietary and lifestyle measures for reducing visceral fat and insulin resistance.
- Address inflammation causes (allergy, infection, heavy metal or chemical toxicity).
- Systemic enzyme therapy.
- Natural anti-inflammatory agents--quercetin, rutin, pine bark extract, grape seed extract (pycnogenol), Boswellia, ginger, EFAs, turmeric, and ice.
- Homeopathics—Traumeel and Zeel.

E. TREAT MITOCHONDRIAL DYSFUNCTION.

CARNITINE HELPS MITOCHONDRIA by transporting fatty acids into the mitochondria, where they are burned to produce energy. This provides energy to your cells and helps you to lose excess fat and maintain an ideal weight. Acetyl-l-carnitine can pass through the blood-brain barrier where it heals the mitochondria inside brain cells. Don't drink alcohol.

- Find out what toxins you are being exposed to now and stop the exposure. Remove the toxins from your body.
- Repair mitochondria with:
  - Lipospheric glutathione.
  - Acetyl-L-Carnitine.
  - Alpha Lipoic Acid.
  - Resveratrol.
  - Pyrroloquinoline quinone (PQQ).
  - Coenzyme Q10 (CoQ10).
  - Vitamin C.
  - Vitamin A.
  - Carnosine.

F. REPAIR CELL DAMAGE.

FAT-SOLUBLE ANTI-OXIDANTS ARE IMPORTANT. They get through the blood-brain barrier and into the cells to get the anti-oxidant activity into the mitochondria to heal the damage done by heavy metals and toxic chemicals.[307] Cell membranes that have been damaged by toxicity may be repaired with certain nutrients.

Scavenge free radicals:

- Vitamin C and E.
- N-Acetyl-Cysteine (NAC).

- Resveratrol.
- Grape-seed extract (pycnogenol).
- Co Q-10.
- Alpha Lipoic Acid and R-Lipoic Acid.
- Acetyl-L-Carnitine.
- Gingko biloba.
- Curcumin.
- Berry pigments—blackberries, blueberries.
- Poly-phenols in green tea.

Repair cell membranes:

- Liposomal Glutathione.
- A phospholipid based repair supplement, like phosphtidylcholine. (Lecithin is phosphatidylcholine and inositol).
- Non-denatured whey protein powder.
- Vitamin D3.
- Vitamin B-12.
- N-Acetyl-Cysteine (NAC).
- Essential Fatty Acids (EFAs).

Eat Cholesterol. Cholesterol helps to keep cell membranes intact and assists with moving needed nutrients in and out of the cell. Make sure you are including plenty of cholesterol-containing foods in your diet. Include butter, avocados, meat, and eggs. The structure of hormones is based on cholesterol.

Cholesterol keeps the immune system and hormones functioning properly. It forms the insulation around nerves.[308] It is essential for your brain to work properly. It stabilizes the neurotransmitters. Without enough cholesterol, a person will become depressed, agitated, and irritable. It is absolutely essential to eat cholesterol-containing foods if you want to optimize metabolism, hormones, and cellular health.

Nature's way to normalize cholesterol levels is simply to eat foods that contain cholesterol like meat, butter, eggs, and shellfish. The body will take what it needs, and then it will switch off cholesterol production. If the cells do not have enough cholesterol, they cannot function properly. If the cells cannot grow properly, they may begin to divide abnormally (cancer).

Heart attacks are related to plaque rupture. Plaque is a sticky substance that is deposited inside the arteries. *Plaque formation is an inflammatory disorder related to toxicity and insulin resistance, not from eating saturated fats.* Studies have shown that eating *excessive* amounts of saturated fats may be related to heart disease.[309]

If you do not eat cholesterol-containing foods, your liver will produce all of the cholesterol that the body needs, unless you are taking statins. But if you rely only on your liver to produce cholesterol, and do not eat cholesterol-containing foods, your liver will *overproduce* cholesterol. If you don't eat cholesterol, the body keeps producing cholesterol, even when there is too much already, thus raising cholesterol far beyond what the body needs.

G. OPTIMIZE NEUROTRANSMITTER LEVELS.

NEUROTRANSMITTERS MAY BE CORRECTED by removing stress, toxins, improper diet, medications, and improper lifestyle. Replacing deficient sex hormones helps to restore neurotransmitter balance. Chronic inflammation is commonly found in people with anxiety, depression, and insomnia. Chronic inflammation affects mood by alternating brain chemistry and hormones. Causes of inflammation (infections, allergies, hypersensitivities, and/or abnormal intestinal permeability) should be evaluated.

1. Serotonin—master neurotransmitter.

Normalizing serotonin levels is the first step in normalizing weight and feeling great. Normal serotonin levels lead to contentment, well-being, focused concentration, and ability to sleep well.

Because serotonin is made from tryptophan, it is important to obtain enough tryptophan. Tryptophan is found in chicken, milk, almonds, cottage cheese, peanuts, shellfish, soy foods, tuna, and turkey. Other important nutrients used to make serotonin are B vitamins, calcium, and magnesium. Serotonin levels will normalize as the metabolism heals by eating a balanced diet. Tryptophan taken at bedtime will aid sleep.

If tryptophan makes you feel bad, or you suspect a chronic inflammatory process, check the results of your kynurenate and quinolinate test, because you may be metabolizing tryptophan into neurotoxic chemicals. If this is the case, look for the cause of the inflammation. Top on the search list would be inflammation in the gut that is caused by infection from bacteria, viruses, parasites, yeast, or leaky gut.

Prescription drugs may help for a while, but they just exacerbate the problem in the long run if the underlying problems are not treated. Many people take antidepressants like Lexapro and Prozac, which are serotonin-reuptake inhibitors (SSRIs). They inhibit the breakdown of serotonin, so the serotonin you have is more potent. That is like having more.

These drugs may make people feel better temporarily because their serotonin levels become elevated, but eventually, if the underlying problem isn't treated, the drugs won't work anymore and create imbalances in the other neurotransmitters. Physicians may then increase the SSRIs, increasing adverse side effects (primarily dry mouth and loss of sexual interest and function), and setting you up for long-term imbalances like restless leg syndrome and severe sleep disturbance.

The solution to serotonin imbalance does not lie in just taking drugs. If you are taking antidepressants, change your lifestyle and find a physician who understands hormonal balance. All too often, cognitive impairment and depression caused by deficient hormones are treated with antidepressants. A poor response to treatment is a primary indication that the proper diagnosis has been overlooked.

If you aren't taking antidepressants and feel depressed, follow the advice in this book with your physician. Antidepressants may be useful or necessary, but usually low-dose antidepressants taken only for short periods will alleviate depression with minimal side effects until hormones are optimized. Inherited and genetically-based major depressions do occur, and antidepressants may be life-saving.

The solution to raise serotonin levels is to eat properly, exercise, manage stress, improve emotional health, avoid the use of stimulants and other drugs, and balance hormones. To achieve normal serotonin levels, it is important to avoid stimulants, drugs of any kind, alcohol, and tobacco, and to eat a diet balanced in proteins, healthy fats, nonstarchy vegetables, and carbohydrates in a level proportionate to energy expenditure. You need adequate proteins and fats to make serotonin and to normalize brain function. Exercise.

Restricting carbohydrates to levels lower than those used for energy production will drop serotonin levels. Low levels lead to depression, apathy, anxiety, lethargy, insomnia, headaches, chronic pain, irritable bowel syndrome, poor attention and focus, and poor memory. This is why those low carbohydrate diets are difficult to follow and one reason why they cause ill health if followed long-term. Low serotonin levels cause cravings for sweets and carbohydrates, which, if eaten, will raise serotonin rapidly. *Often, after following a low-carb or no-carb diet for a while, the urge to eat carbohydrates will rule over the best laid plans and lead to carbohydrate binging.* Alternatives to sweets and simple carbohydrates to increase serotonin include avocados, cottage cheese, egg, pork, wheat germ, and turkey.

Serotonin levels may be repaired with:
- Sufficient, quality sleep.
- 5-HTP raises levels quickly.
- Tryptophan raises levels more slowly.
- Magnesium, calcium, zinc.
- Complex carbohydrates.
- Progesterone.
- Fish oils.
- Pregnenolone.
- Exercise.
- Correcting hormones, especially adrenals.
- SAMe.
- B-6.
- St. John's Wort.
- Melatonin.

2. Acetylcholine.

Acetylcholine levels may be raised with aerobic exercise, testosterone, estrogen, and parathyroid hormones (calcitonin). The most commonly used prescription drug to raise acetylcholine is Aricept, generic name, donepezil. Although beneficial in reversing early symptoms of Alzheimer's, these supplements and drugs won't affect the progression of the disease. When started early, Bioidentical Hormone Replacement Therapy (BHRT) and functional medicine *may* alter the progression.

Foods that will elevate acetylcholine include egg yolk, meat, cereals, milk and cream, and nuts. The supplements, Huperzine A and Vinpocetine, raise acetylcholine and often improve memory. Other supplements that will increase acetylcholine include fish oils, choline, alpha lipoic acid, pantothenic acid, thiamine, B-12, phosphatidylcholine, phosphatidylserine, acetyl-l-carnitine, Taurine, and gingko biloba.

3. Noradrenaline.

Noradrenaline rises with strenuous exercise or pleasure. The enzyme, monoamine oxidase (MAO), will inactivate it. *Bioidentical estradiol in proper levels inhibits MAO, thus elevating mood.*[310] Synthetic progestins stimulate MAO and depress mood.[311] Don't take them. Noradrenaline levels may be supported with the precursor, *N-acetyl tyrosine and tyrosine.* Liposomal cream allows quick absorption across the blood brain barrier.

4. Dopamine.

Foods that will elevate dopamine include all of the foods high in tyrosine and phenylalanine, the precursors to dopamine. They include broccoli, meat, cottage cheese, wheat germ, pork, ricotta cheese, walnuts, chicken, and turkey.

Dopamine levels may be repaired with:
- Weight-bearing exercise.
- Rhodiola Rosea.
- Caffeine.
- CCK.
- DHEA.
- Tyrosine and N-acetyl-tyrosine.

- Methionine.
- Phosphatidylserine.
- Gingko biloba.
- Folic acid.
- Cumin.
- Inositol.
- Testosterone.
- Thyroid.
- Estrogen.

5. GABA.

In women, healthy progesterone levels produce healthy GABA levels, producing calmness. Too much estrogen and too little progesterone (estrogen dominance) may cause women to become too nervous. Low GABA levels cause anxiety and insomnia, which many people medicate with alcohol. A better way to normalize GABA levels is to balance hormones.

Complex carbohydrates produce glutamine, the precursor to GABA. To elevate GABA eat almonds, oats, halibut, rice bran, walnuts, lentils, whole wheat, brown rice, potatoes, and broccoli.

GABA may be repaired with:
- GABA (Oral GABA is poorly absorbed. Try sublingual GABA.)
- Glutamic acid.
- Melatonin.
- Valerian.
- Passion flower.
- Kava.
- Niacinamide.
- Taurine.
- Cinnamon.
- Inositol.
- Theanine.
- CoQ10.
- Prescription drugs—Gabitril (GABA uptake inhibitor).

IMPLEMENT THE SECRET ACTION PLAN!

IF THE TREATMENT PLAN FEELS OVERWHELMING, PRIORITIZE WHAT YOU CAN DO EASILY, AND DO THE THINGS THAT YOU FEEL ARE MOST IMPORTANT. As you add these things into your life, the rest of what you want and need will unfold before you.

Diet – start by adding in, not eliminating. Decide to add in a leafy green vegetable every day. Try cooking kale, onions, and garlic daily.

Start your day with a protein shake. Unsweetened whey-based protein powder is well-tolerated by most of us and tastes sweet. Avoid any protein powder with additives – sucrose or sugar especially. Add fresh or frozen organic fruits, powdered vitamins and supplements. Some high-nutrition powders include brewer's yeast, lecithin, Spirulina, chlorella, Vitamin C, and minerals. Unrefined coconut oil will add medium chain triglycerides.

You can save 30% or more by buying powders over tablets or capsules. Powders are absorbed much better than tablets, especially if you have digestive disorders. Buying online may save up to another 30%. Avoid buying expensive combination products. Buy the separate ingredients in powder form and save 50-90% over the expensive combination products. Add snacks to your diet every four hours with fifteen grams of carbohydrate.

Exercise. Add walking fifteen minutes a day. Start with seven and one-half minutes out and seven and one-half minutes back. Add one minute a week and never miss a day. Find exercise that you like and stick with it.

When you walk, try to be present in the moment. You will find you will start playing the tapes that run through your mind. Just turn them off and keep repeating the words, "Be here now." Feel your life force, your consciousness; feel it here in this place; feel it here in this moment.

De-stress. Add prayer or meditation into your day. Turn your attention inward for fifteen minutes a day. On the inhale bring light and energy in through the top of your head, down the front of the spine, and down the inside of the legs. On the exhale let go of ALL of the negative thoughts that do not serve you as you imagine the energy coming back up through the inside of your legs, up the back of the spine, and out through the top of your head. As you let go of all of the negativity, look for a feeling of gratitude for all the blessings of your life.

Detoxify. Start reading the label and ingredients of everything you buy. Don't buy anything with preservatives, artificial color or flavors, high fructose corn syrup, or hydrogenated vegetable oils. If you do this you, will find that you can't buy about 75% of what is in the major grocery chain stores. If we all start caring for our health and what we eat, the food manufacturers will change what they are offering us.

Good luck in your efforts to heal your sick metabolism and lose toxic belly fat. It isn't an easy task in this toxic world that we live in. But the payoff in your health is well worth it!

By carefully following the secret action plan, you will be able to eliminate toxic belly fat, get healthier and balance your hormones. You will:

- *Look great!*
- *Feel great!*
- *Lose weight!*
- *Have better sex!*

For more information about how to implement the secret action plan, go to Dr.Hormone.org.

REFERENCES

[1] Fauci AS, Kasper DL, Longo DL, Braunwald E, Hauser SL, Jameson JL, Loscalzo J. *Harrison's Principles of Internal Medicine. 17th Edition.* McGraw Hill. New York, New York. 2008. p.463.

[2] Ganong WF. *Review of Medical Physiology. 22nd edition.* McGraw Hill. Boston, MA. 2005. p.346-7.

[3] Ganong WF. *Review of Medical Physiology. 22nd edition.* McGraw Hill. Boston, MA. 2005. p.348.

[4] Moyad MA. Fad diets and obesity--Part IV: Low-carbohydrate vs. low-fat diets. *Urol Nurs. 2005 Feb;25(1):67-70.*

[5] Ferriby LL, Knutsen JS, Harris M, et al. Evaluation of PCDD/F and dioxin-like PCB serum concentration data from the 2001-2002 National Health and Nutrition Examination Survey of the United States population. *J Expo Sci Environ Epidemiol. Jul 2007;17(4):358-371.*

[6] Krewski D, Andersen ME, Mantus E, Zeise L. Toxicity testing in the 21st century: implications for human health risk assessment. *Risk Anal. Apr 2009;29(4):474-479.*

[7] Slotkin TA. Does early-life exposure to organophosphate insecticides lead to prediabetes and obesity? *Reprod Toxicol. 2011 Apr;31(3):297-301.*

[8] Pelltier C, Doucet E, Imbeault P, Tremblay A. Associations between weight loss-induced changes in plasma organochlorine concentrations, serum T(3) concentration, and resting metabolic rate. *Toxicol Sci. May 2002;67(1):46-51.*

[9] Hue O, Marcotte J, Berrigan F, et al. Increased plasma levels of toxic pollutants accompanying weight loss induced by hypocaloric diet or by bariatric surgery. *Obes Surg. Sep 2006;16(9):1145-1154.*

[10] Paustenbach D GD. Biomonitoring: is body burden relevant to public health? *Regul Toxicol Pharmacol. 2006;44(3):249-261.*

[11] Ruzzin J, Petersen R, Meugnier E, Madsen L, Lock EJ, Lillefosse H, Ma T, Pesenti S, Sonne SB, Marstrand TT, Malde MK, Du ZY, Chavey C, Fajas L, Lundebye AK, Brand CL, Vidal H, Kristiansen K, Frøyland L. Persistent organic pollutant exposure leads to insulin resistance syndrome. *Environ Health Perspect. 2010 Apr;118(4):465-71.*

[12] Crinnion WJ. Do environmental toxicants contribute to allergy and asthma? *Altern Med Rev. 2012 Mar;17(1):6-18.*

[13] Schug TT, Janesick A, Blumberg B, Heindel JJ. Endocrine disrupting chemicals and disease susceptibility. *J Steroid Biochem Mol Biol. 2011 Nov;127(3-5):204-15.*

[14] Judson RS, Martin MT, Egeghy P, Gangwal S, Reif DM, Kothiya P, Wolf M, Cathey T, Transue T, Smith D, Vail J, Frame A, Mosher S, Cohen Hubal EA, Richard AM. Aggregating Data for Computational Toxicology Applications: The U.S.Environmental Protection Agency (EPA) Aggregated Computational Toxicology Resource (ACToR) System. *Int J Mol Sci. 2012;13(2):1805-31.*

[15] -Heel. *Biotherapeutic Index Ordinatio Antihomotixica et Materia Medica.* Biologishch Heilmittel Heel GmbH, Dr.-Reckeweg-StraBe 2-4 96532 Konkordia Druck GmbH, Buhl. Baden-Baden Germany. 1986. p. 11.

[16] Crinnion WJ. Environmental medicine, part 4: pesticides – biologically persistent and ubiquitous toxins. *Altern Med Rev. 2000 Oct;5(5):432-47.*

[17] Kohler BA, Ward E, McCarthy BJ, Schymura MJ, Ries LA, Eheman C, Jemal A, Anderson RN, Ajani UA, Edwards BK. Annual report to the nation on the status of cancer, 1975-2007, featuring tumors of the brain and other nervous system. *J Natl Cancer Inst. 2011 May 4;103(9):714-36.*

[18] Kogevinas M, Villanueva CM, Font-Ribera L, Liviac D, Bustamante M, Espinoza F, Nieuwenhuijsen MJ, Espinosa A, Fernandez P, DeMarini DM, Grimalt JO, Grummt T, Marcos R. Genotoxic effects in swimmers exposed to disinfection by-products in indoor swimming pools. *Environ Health Perspect. 2010 Nov;118(11):1531-7.*

[19] Villanueva CM, Cantor KP, Grimalt JO, Malats N, Silverman D, Tardon A, Garcia-Closas R, Serra C, Carrato A, Castaño-Vinyals G, Marcos R, Rothman N, Real FX, Dosemeci M, Kogevinas M. Bladder cancer and exposure to water disinfection by-products through ingestion, bathing, showering, and swimming in pools. *Am J Epidemiol. 2007 Jan 15;165(2):148-56.*

[20] Morris RD. Drinking water and cancer. *Environ Health Perspect. 1995 Nov;103 Suppl 8:225-31. Review.*

[21] Monroe RK, Halvorsen SW. Environmental toxicants inhibit neuronal Jak tyrosine kinase by mitochondrial disruption. *Neurotoxicology. 2009 Jul;30(4):589-98.*

[22] Stephany RW. Hormones in meat: different approaches in the EU and in the USA. *APMIS Suppl. 2001;(103):S357-63; discussion S363-4.*

[23] Bustnes JO, Lie E, Herzke D, Dempster T, Bjørn PA, Nygård T, Uglem I. Salmon Farms as a Source of Organohalogenated Contaminants in Wild Fish. *Environ Sci Technol. 2010 Nov 15;44(22):8736-8743.*

[24] Nierenberg D. Rethinking the global meat industry. *State of the World 2006; Worldwatch Institute: p.26.*

[25] Reece RL, Barr DA, Forsyth WM, Scott PC. Investigations of toxicity episodes involving chemotherapeutic agents in Victorian poultry and pigeons. *Avian Dis.1985 Oct-Dec;29(4):1239-51.*

[26] Nachman KE, Raber G, Francesconi KA, Navas-Acien A, Love DC. Arsenic species in poultry feather meal. *Sci Total Environ. 2012 Feb 15;417-418:183-8.*

[27] Otleş S, Cağindi O. Health importance of arsenic in drinking water and food. *Environ Geochem Health. 2010 Aug;32(4):367-71.*

[28] Christen K. Chickens, manure, and arsenic. *Environ Sci Technol. 2001 May1;35(9):184A-185A.*

[29] Ibrahim MM, Fjære E, Lock EJ, Naville D, Amlund H, Meugnier E, Le Magueresse Battistoni B, Frøyland L, Madsen L, Jessen N, Lund S, Vidal H, Ruzzin J. Chronic consumption of farmed salmon containing persistent organic pollutants causes insulin resistance and obesity in mice. *PLoS One. 2011;6(9):e25170.*

[30] Foran JA, Carpenter DO, Hamilton MC, Knuth BA, Schwager SJ. Risk-based consumption advice for farmed Atlantic and wild Pacific salmon contaminated with dioxins and dioxin-like compounds. *Environ Health Perspect. 2005 May;113(5):552-6.*

[31] Nijman NM, Oosterhuis JA, van Bijsterveld OP, Baart de la Faille H, Suurmond D. [Canthaxanthin retinopathy]. *Klin Monbl Augenheilkd. 1989 Jan;194(1):48-51. German.*

[32] Sunderland EM. Mercury exposure from domestic and imported estuarine and marine fish in the U.S. seafood market. *Environ Health Perspect. 2007Feb;115(2):235-42.*

[33] Tate PL, Bibb R, Larcom LL. Milk stimulates growth of prostate cancer cells in culture. *Nutr Cancer. 2011 Nov;63(8):1361-6.*

[34] Costa TE, Marin VA. Labeling of food containing genetically modified organisms: international policies and Brazilian legislation. *Cien Saude Colet.2011 Aug;16(8):3571-82.*

[35] de Sitter H, Peters PW. Biotechnology, especially genetic modification, and legislation. *Tijdschr Diergeneeskd. 2002 May 15;127(10):322-30.*

[36] Louz D, Bergmans HE, Loos BP, Hoeben RC. Cross-species transfer of viruses: implications for the use of viral vectors in biomedical research, gene therapy and as live-virus vaccines. *J Gene Med. 2005 Oct;7(10):1263-74.*

[37] Poulsen LK. Allergy assessment of foods or ingredients derived from biotechnology, gene-modified organisms, or novel foods. *Mol Nutr Food Res. 2004 Nov;48(6):413-23.*

[38] Cantani A. Benefits and concerns associated with biotechnology-derived foods: can additional research reduce children health risks? *Eur Rev Med Pharmacol Sci. 2006 Jul-Aug;10(4):197-206.*

[39] Jurewicz J, Hanke W, Radwan M, Bonde JP. Environmental factors and semen quality. *Int J Occup Med Environ Health. 2009;22(4):305-29.*

[40] Focke F, Schuermann D, Kuster N, Schär P (November 2009). DNA fragmentation in human fibroblasts under extremely low frequency electromagnetic field exposure. *Mutation Research 683 (1-2): 74–83.*

[41] Sohrabi MR, Tarjoman T, Abadi A, Yavari P. Living near overhead high voltage transmission power lines as a risk factor for childhood acute lymphoblastic leukemia: a case-control study. *Asian Pac J Cancer Prev. 2010;11(2):423-7.*

[42] The probability of developing brain tumours among users of cellular telephones (scientific information to the decision of the International Agency for Research on Cancer (IARC) announced on May 31, 2011). *Radiats Biol Radioecol. 2011 Sep-Oct;51(5):633-8.*

[43] Stam R. Electromagnetic fields and the blood-brain barrier. *Brain Res Rev. 2010 Oct 5;65(1):80-97.*

[44] Carpenter DO. Electromagnetic fields and cancer: the cost of doing nothing. Rev Environ Health. *2010 Jan-Mar;25(1):75-80.*

[45] Zimmerman MR, Trinkaus E, LeMay M, Aufderheide AC, Reyman TA, Marrocco GR, Ortel RW, Benitez JT, Laughlin WS, Horne PD, Schultes RE, Coughlin EA. The paleopathology of an Aleutian mummy. *Arch Pathol Lab Med. 1981 Dec;105(12):638-41.*

[46] Zimmerman MR. An experimental study of mummification pertinent to the antiquity of cancer. *Cancer. 1977 Sep;40(3):1358-62.*

[47] Martínez-García MJ, Moreno JM, Moreno-Clavel J, Vergara N, García-Sánchez A, Guillamón A, Portí M, Moreno-Grau S. Heavy metals in human bones in different historical epochs. *Sci Total Environ. 2005 Sep 15;348(1-3):51-72.*

[48] Irigaray P, Newby JA, Clapp R, Hardell L, Howard V, Montagnier L, Epstein S, Belpomme D. Lifestyle-related factors and environmental agents causing cancer: an overview. *Biomed Pharmacother. 2007 Dec;61(10):640-58.*

[49] Lichtenstein P, Holm NV, Verkasalo PK, Iliadou A, Kaprio J, Koskenvuo M, Pukkala E, Skytthe A, Hemminki K. Environmental and heritable factors in the causation of cancer—analysis of cohorts of twins from Sweden, Denmark, and Finland. *N Engl J Med 2000;343(2):78-85.*

[50] Anand P, Kunnumakkara AB, Sundaram C, Harikumar KB, Tharakan ST, Lai OS, Sung B, Aggarwal BB. Cancer is a preventable disease that requires major lifestyle changes. *Pharm Res. 2008 Sep;25(9):2097-116.*

[51] Soto AM, Sonnenschein C. Environmental causes of cancer: endocrine disruptors as carcinogens. *Nat Rev Endocrinol. 2010 Jul;6(7):363-70.*

[52] Bradlow HL, Davis DL, Lin G, Sepkovic D, Tiwari R. Effects of pesticides on the ratio of 16 alpha/2-hydroxyestrone: a biologic marker of breast cancer risk. *Environ Health Perspect. 1995 Oct;103 Suppl 7:147-50.*

[53] Wetherill YB, Petre CE, Monk KR, Puga A, Knudsen KE. The xenoestrogen bisphenol A induces inappropriate androgen receptor activation and mitogenesis in prostatic adenocarcinoma cells. *Mol Cancer Ther. 2002*

May;1(7):515-24.

[54] De Flora S, Micale RT, La Maestra S, Izzotti A, D'Agostini F, Camoirano A, Davoli SA, Troglio MG, Rizzi F, Davalli P, Bettuzzi S. Upregulation of clusterin in prostate and DNA damage in spermatozoa from bisphenol A-treated rats and formation of DNA adducts in cultured human prostatic cells. *Toxicol Sci. 2011 Jul;122(1):45-51.*

[55] Crinnion WJ. Maternal levels of xenobiotics that affect fetal development and childhood health. *Altern Med Rev. 2009 Sep;14(3):212-22.*

[56] Isaac CP, Sivakumar A, Kumar CR. Lead levels in breast milk, blood plasma and intelligence quotient: a health hazard for women and infants. *Bull Environ Contam Toxicol. 2012 Feb;88(2):145-9.*

[57] Calafat AM, Slakman AR, Silva MJ, Herbert AR, Needham LL. Automated solid phase extraction and quantitative analysis of human milk for 13 phthalate metabolites. *J Chromatogr B Analyt Technol Biomed Life Sci. 2004 Jun 5;805(1):49-56.*

[58] Cressey PJ, Vannoort RW. Pesticide content of infant formulae and weaning foods available in New Zealand. *Food Addit Contam. 2003 Jan;20(1):57-64.*

[59] Massey-Stokes M, Lanning B. Childhood cancer and environmental toxins: the debate continues. *Fam Community Health. 2002 Jan;24(4):27-38.*

[60] Forouzanfar MH, Foreman KJ, Delossantos AM, Lozano R, Lopez AD, Murray CJ, Naghavi M. Breast and cervical cancer in 187 countries between 1980 and 2010: a systematic analysis. *Lancet. 2011 Oct 22;378(9801):1461-84.*

[61] Crinnion WJ. Environmental medicine, part one: the human burden of environmental toxins and their common health effects. *Altern Med Rev. 2000 Feb;5(1):52-63.*

[62] Bethwaite PB, Pearce N, Fraser J. Cancer risks in painters: study based on the New Zealand Cancer Registry. *Br J Ind Med. 1990 Nov;47(11):742-6.*

[63] Feldman RG. Central and peripheral nervous system effects of metals: a survey. *Acta Neurol Scand Suppl. 1982;92:143-66.*

[64] Koedrith P, Seo YR. Advances in carcinogenic metal toxicity and potential molecular markers. *Int J Mol Sci. 2011;12(12):9576-95.*

[65] Houston MC. Role of mercury toxicity in hypertension, cardiovascular disease, and stroke. *J Clin Hypertens (Greenwich). 2011 Aug;13(8):621-7.*

[66] Houston MC. The role of mercury and cadmium heavy metals in vascular disease, hypertension, coronary heart disease, and myocardial infarction. *Altern Ther Health Med. 2007 Mar-Apr;13(2):S128-33.*

[67] Yoshizuka M, Mori N, Hamasaki K, Tanaka I, Yokoyama M, Hara K, Doi Y, Umezu Y, Araki H, Sakamoto Y, et al. Cadmium toxicity in the thyroid gland of pregnant rats. *Exp Mol Pathol. 1991 Aug;55(1):97-104.*

[68] Whaley-Connell A, McCullough PA, Sowers JR. The role of oxidative stress in the metabolic syndrome. *Rev Cardiovasc Med. 2011;12(1):21-9.*

[69] Han Wei, Dan Wei, Shuo Yi, Fang Zhang, Wenjun Ding. Oxidative stress induced by urban fine particles in cultured EA.hy926 cells. *Hum Exp Toxicol. 2011 Jul;30(7):579-90.*

[70] Ciolino HP, Levine RL. Modification of proteins in endothelial cell death during oxidative stress. *Free Radic Biol Med. 1997;22(7):1277-82*

[71] Kaji T, Fujiwara Y, Hoshino M, Yamamoto C, Sakamoto M, Kozuka H. Inhibitory effect of lead on the proliferation of cultured vascular endothelial cells. *Toxicology. 1995 Jan 6;95(1-3):87-92.*

[72] Belyaeva EA, Dymkowska D, Wieckowski MR, Wojtczak L. Mitochondria as an important target in heavy metal toxicity in rat hepatoma AS-30D cells. *Toxicol Appl Pharmacol. 2008 Aug 15;231(1):34-42.*

[73] Houston MC. Role of mercury toxicity in hypertension, cardiovascular disease, and stroke. *J Clin Hypertens (Greenwich). 2011 Aug;13(8):621-7.*

[74] Su B, Wang X, Zheng L, Perry G, Smith MA, Zhu X. Abnormal mitochondrial dynamics and neurodegenerative diseases. *Biochim Biophys Acta. 2010 Jan;1802(1):135-42.*

[75] Crinnion WJ. Polychlorinated biphenyls: persistent pollutants with immunological, neurological, and endocrinological consequences. *Altern Med Rev. 2011 Mar;16(1):5-13.*

[76] Fukuyama T, Tajima Y, Ueda H, Hayashi K, Shutoh Y, Harada T, Kosaka T. Apoptosis in immunocytes induced by several types of pesticides. *J Immunotoxicol. 2010 Mar;7(1):39-56.*

[77] Kaji T. [Cell biology of heavy metal toxicity in vascular tissue]. *Yakugaku Zasshi. 2004 Mar;124(3):113-20.*

[78] Bautista LE, Stein JH, Morgan BJ, Stanton N, Young T, Nieto FJ. Association of blood and hair mercury with blood pressure and vascular reactivity. *WMJ. 2009 Aug;108(5):250-2.*

[79] Bertossi M, Girolamo F, Errede M, Virgintino D, Elia G, Ambrosi L, Roncali L. Effects of methylmercury on the microvasculature of the developing brain. *Neurotoxicology. 2004 Sep;25(5):849-57.*

[80] Kaji T, Fujiwara Y, Hoshino M, Yamamoto C, Sakamoto M, Kozuka H. Inhibitory effect of lead on the proliferation of cultured vascular endothelial cells. *Toxicology. 1995 Jan 6;95(1-3):87-92.*

[81] Darbre PD. Metalloestrogens: an emerging class of inorganic xenoestrogens with potential to add to the oestrogenic

burden of the human breast. *J Appl Toxicol. 2006 May-Jun;26(3):191-7.*

[82] Gallagher CM, Meliker JR. Mercury and thyroid autoantibodies in U.S. women, *NHANES 2007-2008. Environ Int. 2012 Apr;40:39-43.*

[83] Crinnion WJ. Environmental medicine, part three: long-term effects of chronic low-dose mercury exposure. *Altern Med Rev. 2000 Jun;5(3):209-23.*

[84] Gerstenberger SL, Martinson A, Kramer JL. An evaluation of mercury concentrations in three brands of canned tuna. *Environ Toxicol Chem. 2010 Feb;29(2):237-42.*

[85] Drum DA. Are toxic biometals destroying your children's future? *Biometals. 2009 Oct;22(5):697-700.*

[86] Barocas R, Weiss B. Behavioral assessment of lead intoxication in children. *Environ Health Perspect. 1974 May;7:47-52.*

[87] Needleman HL, Riess JA, Tobin MJ, Biesecker GE, Greenhouse JB. Bone lead levels and delinquent behavior. *JAMA. 1996 Feb 7;275(5):363-9.*

[88] Pezzotti A, Kraft P, Hankinson SE, Hunter DJ, Buring J, Cox DG. The mitochondrial A10398G polymorphism, interaction with alcohol consumption, and breast cancer risk. *PLoS One. 2009;4(4):e5356.*

[89] Wright YL, *Fat Loss Secrets that Really Work--Balance Your Hormones: Insulin, Estrogen, Progesterone, Testosterone, Thyroid, Cortisol, and DHEA!* Lulu.com. 2012. p.32.

[90] Laidlaw MA, Taylor MP. Potential for childhood lead poisoning in the inner cities of Australia due to exposure to lead in soil dust. *Environ Pollut. 2011 Jan;159(1):1-9.*

[91] Julin B, Wolk A, Bergkvist L, Bottai M, Akesson A. Dietary cadmium exposure and risk of postmenopausal breast cancer: a population-based prospective cohort study. *Cancer Res. 2012 Mar 15;72(6):1459-66.*

[92] Sahmoun AE, Case LD, Jackson SA, Schwartz GG. Cadmium and prostate cancer: a critical epidemiologic analysis. *Cancer Invest. 2005;23(3):256-63.*

[93] Julin B, Wolk A, Bergkvist L, Bottai M, Akesson A. Dietary cadmium exposure and risk of postmenopausal breast cancer: a population-based prospective cohort study. *Cancer Res. 2012 Mar 15;72(6):1459-66.*

[94] Kaji T, Suzuki M, Yamamoto C, Mishima A, Sakamoto M, Kozuka H. Severe damage of cultured vascular endothelial cell monolayer after simultaneous exposure to cadmium and lead. *Arch Environ Contam Toxicol. 1995 Feb;28(2):168-72.*

[95] Kaji T, Mishima A, Yamamoto C, Sakamoto M, Kozuka H. Zinc protection against cadmium-induced destruction of the monolayer of cultured vascular endothelial cells. *Toxicol Lett. 1993 Mar;66(3):247-55.*

[96] Needleman HL, Riess JA, Tobin MJ, Biesecker GE, Greenhouse JB. Bone lead levels and delinquent behavior. *JAMA. 1996 Feb 7;275(5):363-9.*

[97] Frisardi V, Solfrizzi V, Capurso C, Kehoe PG, Imbimbo BP, Santamato A, Dellegrazie F, Seripa D, Pilotto A, Capurso A, Panza F. Aluminum in the diet and Alzheimer's disease: from current epidemiology to possible disease-modifying treatment. *J Alzheimers Dis. 2010;20(1):17-30.*

[98] Exley C. Does antiperspirant use increase the risk of aluminium-related disease, including Alzheimer's disease? *Mol Med Today. 1998 Mar;4(3):107-9.*

[99] Gondal MA, Seddigi ZS, Nasr MM, Gondal B. Spectroscopic detection of health hazardous contaminants in lipstick using Laser Induced Breakdown Spectroscopy. *J Hazard Mater. 2010 Mar 15;175(1-3):726-32.*

[100] McGrath KG. An earlier age of breast cancer diagnosis related to more frequent use of antiperspirants/deodorants and underarm shaving. *Eur J Cancer Prev. 2003 Dec;12(6):479-85.*

[101] McGrath KG. Apocrine sweat gland obstruction by antiperspirants allowing transdermal absorption of cutaneous generated hormones and pheromones as a link to the observed incidence rates of breast and prostate cancer in the 20th century. *Med Hypotheses. 2009 Jun;72(6):665-74.*

[102] Lasky T, Sun W, Kadry A, Hoffman MK. Mean total arsenic concentrations in chicken 1989-2000 and estimated exposures for consumers of chicken. *Environ Health Perspect. 2004 Jan;112(1):18-21.*

[103] Morris RD. Drinking water and cancer. *Environ Health Perspect. 1995 Nov;103 Suppl 8:225-31. Review.*

[104] Heck JE, Andrew AS, Onega T, Rigas JR, Jackson BP, Karagas MR, Duell EJ. Lung cancer in a U.S. population with low to moderate arsenic exposure. *Environ Health Perspect. 2009 Nov;117(11):1718-23.*

[105] Leonardi G, Vahter M, Clemens F, Goessler W, Gurzau E, Hemminki K, Hough R, Koppova K, Kumar R, Rudnai P, Surdu S, Fletcher T. Arsenic and Basal Cell Carcinoma in Areas of Hungary, Romania, and Slovakia: A Case-Control Study. *Environ Health Perspect. 2012 Jan 31.*

[106] Radosavljević V, Jakovljević B. Arsenic and bladder cancer: observations and suggestions. *J Environ Health. 2008 Oct;71(3):40-2.*

[107] Kádas I, Balázs L, Pár A, Barna K. Angiosarcoma of the liver following brief arsenic therapy. *Zentralbl Allg Pathol. 1985;130(6):539-43.*

[108] Smith AH, Hopenhayn-Rich C, Bates MN, Goeden HM, Hertz-Picciotto I, Duggan HM, Wood R, Kosnett MJ, Smith MT. Cancer risks from arsenic in drinking water. *Environ Health Perspect. 1992 Jul;97:259-67.*

[109] Singh KP, Kumari R, Treas J, DuMond JW. Chronic exposure to arsenic causes increased cell survival, DNA damage, and increased expression of mitochondrial transcription factor A (mtTFA) in human prostate epithelial cells. *Chem Res Toxicol. 2011 Mar 21;24(3):340-9.*

[110] Su CC, Lu JL, Tsai KY, Lian IeB. Reduction in arsenic intake from water has different impacts on lung cancer and bladder cancer in an arseniasis endemic area in Taiwan. *Cancer Causes Control. 2011 Jan;22(1):101-8.*

[111] Yu HS, Liao WT, Chai CY. Arsenic carcinogenesis in the skin. *J Biomed Sci. 2006 Sep;13(5):657-66.*

[112] Walker P, Rhubart-Berg P, McKenzie S, Kelling K, Lawrence RS. Public health implications of meat production and consumption. *Public Health Nutr. Jun 2005;8(4):348-356.*

[113] Schell LM, Gallo MV, Ravenscroft J, DeCaprio AP. Persistent organic pollutants and anti-thyroid peroxidase levels in Akwesasne Mohawk young adults. *Environ Res. Jan 2009;109(1):86-92.*

[114] Salay E, Garabrant D. Polychlorinated biphenyls and thyroid hormones in adults: a systematic review appraisal of epidemiological studies. *Chemosphere. Mar 2009;74(11):1413-1419.*

[115] Charlier C, Desaive C, Plomteux G. Human exposure to endocrine disrupters: consequences of gastroplasty on plasma concentration of toxic pollutants. *Int J Obes Relat Metab Disord. Nov 2002;26(11):1465-1468.*

[116] Imbeault P, Chevrier J, Dewailly E, et al. Increase in plasma pollutant levels in response to weight loss is associated with the reduction of fasting insulin levels in men but not in women. *Metabolism. Apr 2002;51(4):482-486.*

[117] Pelletier C, Imbeault P, Tremblay A. Energy balance and pollution by organochlorines and polychlorinated biphenyls. *Obes Rev. Feb 2003;4(1):17-24.*

[118] Mullerova D, Kopecky J, Matejkova D, et al. Negative association between plasma levels of adiponectin and polychlorinated biphenyl 153 in obese women under non-energy-restrictive regime. *Int J Obes (Lond). Dec 2008;32(12):1875-1878.*

[119] Pelltier C, Doucet E, Imbeault P, Tremblay A. Associations between weight loss-induced changes in plasma organochlorine concentrations, serum T(3) concentration, and resting metabolic rate. *Toxicol Sci. May 2002;67(1):46-51.*

[120] Villanueva CM, Cantor KP, Grimalt JO, Castaño-Vinyals G, Malats N, Silverman D, Tardon A, Garcia-Closas R, Serra C, Carrato A, Rothman N, Real FX, Dosemeci M, Kogevinas M. Assessment of lifetime exposure to trihalomethanes through different routes. *Occup Environ Med. 2006 Apr;63(4):273-7.*

[121] Wiest L. Chemical peels in aesthetic dermatology. *Hautarzt. 2004 Jul;55(7):611-20. Review.*

[122] Coplan MJ, Patch SC, Masters RD, Bachman MS. Confirmation of and explanations for elevated blood lead and other disorders in children exposed to water disinfection and fluoridation chemicals. *Neurotoxicology. 2007 Sep;28(5):1032-42.*

[123] Haojun Z, Yaoling W, Ke Z, Jin L, Junling W. Effects of NaF on the expression of intracellular Ca(2+) fluxes and apoptosis and the antagonism of taurine in murine neuron. *Toxicol Mech Methods. 2012 May;22(4):305-8.*

[124] Stackelberg PE, Furlong ET, Meyer MT, Zaugg SD, Henderson AK, Reissman DB. Persistence of pharmaceutical compounds and other organic wastewater contaminants in a conventional drinking-water-treatment plant. *Sci Total Environ. 2004 Aug 15;329(1-3):99-113.*

[125] Tedeschi LG. Dioxin. A case in point. Am J Forensic Med Pathol. *1980 Jun;1(2):145-8.*

[126] Baris RD, Cohen SZ, Barnes NL, Lam J, Ma Q. Quantitative analysis of over 20 years of golf course monitoring studies. *Environ Toxicol Chem. 2010 Jun;29(6):1224-36.*

[127] McLeod CG Jr, Singer AW, Harrington DG. Acute neuropathology in soman poisoned rats. *Neurotoxicology. 1984 Summer;5(2):53-7.*

[128] Garg UK, Pal AK, Jha GJ, Jadhao SB. Pathophysiological effects of chronic toxicity with synthetic pyrethroid, organophosphate and chlorinated pesticides on bone health of broiler chicks. *Toxicol Pathol. 2004 May Jun;32(3):364-9.*

[129] Norimoto K, Kiuchi K, Morikawa M, Inoue Y, Kosaka J, Inoue M, Kishimoto T. Parkinsonism with multiple cysts in the bilateral striata. *Psychogeriatrics. 2011 Sep;11(3):166-70.*

[130] Woodward G. Autism and Parkinson's disease. *Med Hypotheses. 2001 Feb;56(2):246-9.*

[131] Roberts EM, English PB, Grether JK, Windham GC, Somberg L, Wolff C. Maternal residence near agricultural pesticide applications and autism spectrum disorders among children in the California Central Valley. *Environ Health Perspect. 2007 Oct;115(10):1482-9.*

[132] Kurt TL. Epidemiological association in US veterans between Gulf War illness and exposures to anticholinesterases. *Toxicol Lett. 1998 Dec 28;102-103:523-6.*

[133] Haley RW, Kurt TL. Self-reported exposure to neurotoxic chemical combinations in the Gulf War. A cross-sectional epidemiologic study. *JAMA. 1997 Jan 15;277(3):231-7.*

[134] Sepkovic DW, Bradlow HL. Estrogen hydroxylation--the good and the bad. *Ann N Y Acad Sci. 2009 Feb;1155:57-67.*

[135] Hombach-Klonisch S, Pocar P, Kauffold J, Klonisch T. Dioxin exerts anti-estrogenic actions in a novel dioxin-responsive telomerase-immortalized epithelial cell line of the porcine oviduct (TERT-OPEC). *Toxicol Sci. 2006 Apr;90(2):519-28.*

[136] van Duursen MB, Sanderson JT, van der Bruggen M, van der Linden J, van den Berg M. Effects of several dioxin-like compounds on estrogen metabolism in the malignant MCF-7 and nontumorigenic MCF-10A human mammary epithelial cell lines. *Toxicol Appl Pharmacol. 2003 Aug 1;190(3):241-50.*

[137] Tranfo G, Caporossi L, Paci E, Aragona C, Romanzi D, De Carolis C, De Rosa M, Capanna S, Papaleo B, Pera A. Urinary phthalate monoesters concentration in couples with infertility problems. *Toxicol Lett. 2011 Dec 16.*

[138] Lithner D, Nordensvan I, Dave G. Comparative acute toxicity of leachates from plastic products made of polypropylene, polyethylene, PVC, acrylonitrile-butadiene-styrene, and epoxy to Daphnia magna. *Environ Sci Pollut Res Int. 2011 Dec 20.*

[139] Hsieh HI, Chen PC, Wong RH, Du CL, Chang YY, Wang JD, Cheng TJ. Mortality from liver cancer and leukaemia among polyvinyl chloride workers in Taiwan: an updated study. *Occup Environ Med. 2011 Feb;68(2):120-5.*

[140] Shen C, Chen Y, Huang S, Wang Z, Yu C, Qiao M, Xu Y, Setty K, Zhang J, Zhu Y, Lin Q. Dioxin-like compounds in agricultural soils near e-waste recycling sites from Taizhou area, China: chemical and bioanalytical characterization. *Environ Int. 2009 Jan;35(1):50-5.*

[141] Erler C, Novak J. Bisphenol a exposure: human risk and health policy. *J Pediatr Nurs. 2010 Oct;25(5):400-7.*

[142] Seité S, Moyal D, Verdier MP, Hourseau C, Fourtanier A. Accumulated p53protein and UVA protection level of sunscreens. *Photodermatol Photoimmunol Photomed. 2000 Feb;16(1):3-9.*

[143] Petković J, Zegura B, Stevanović M, Drnovšek N, Uskoković D, Novak S, Filipič M. DNA damage and alterations in expression of DNA damage responsive genes induced by TiO2 nanoparticles in human hepatoma HepG2 cells. *Nanotoxicology. 2011 Sep;5(3):341-53.*

[144] Trouiller B, Reliene R, Westbrook A, Solaimani P, Schiestl RH. Titanium dioxide nanoparticles induce DNA damage and genetic instability in vivo in mice. *Cancer Res. 2009 Nov 15;69(22):8784-9.*

[145] Msiska Z, Pacurari M, Mishra A, Leonard SS, Castranova V, Vallyathan V. DNA double-strand breaks by asbestos, silica, and titanium dioxide: possible biomarker of carcinogenic potential? *Am J Respir Cell Mol Biol. 2010 Aug;43(2):210-9.*

[146] Buzea C, Pacheco II, Robbie K. Nanomaterials and nanoparticles: sources and toxicity. *Biointerphases. 2007 Dec;2(4):MR17-71.*

[147] Nakagawa Y, Suzuki T. Metabolism of 2-hydroxy-4-methoxybenzophenone in isolated rat hepatocytes and xenoestrogenic effects of its metabolites on MCF-7 human breast cancer cells. *Chem Biol Interact. 2002 Feb 20;139(2):115-28.*

[148] Schlumpf M, Cotton B, Conscience M, Haller V, Steinmann B, Lichtensteiger W. In vitro and in vivo estrogenicity of UV screens. *Environ Health Perspect. 2001 Mar;109(3):239-44.*

[149] Calafat AM, Wong LY, Ye X, Reidy JA, Needham LL. Concentrations of the sunscreen agent benzophenone-3 in residents of the United States: National Health and Nutrition Examination Survey 2003--2004. *Environ Health Perspect. 2008 Jul;116(7):893-7.*

[150] Xu C, Green A, Parisi A, Parsons PG. Photosensitization of the sunscreen octyl p-dimethylaminobenzoate by UVA in human melanocytes but not in keratinocytes. *Photochem Photobiol. 2001 Jun;73(6):600-4.*

[151] Cook N, Freeman S. Photosensitive dermatitis due to sunscreen allergy in a child. *Australas J Dermatol. 2002 May;43(2):133-5.*

[152] Cook N, Freeman S. Report of 19 cases of photoallergic contact dermatitis to sunscreens seen at the Skin and Cancer Foundation. *Australas J Dermatol. 2001 Nov;42(4):257-9.*

[153] Katsarou A, Makris M, Zarafonitis G, Lagogianni E, Gregoriou S, Kalogeromitros D. Photoallergic contact dermatitis: the 15-year experience of a tertiary reference center in a sunny Mediterranean city. *Int J Immunopathol Pharmacol.2008 Jul-Sep;21(3):725-7.*

[154] Fischer T, Bergström K. Evaluation of customers' complaints about sunscreen cosmetics sold by the Swedish pharmaceutical company. *Contact Dermatitis. 1991 Nov;25(5):319-22.*

[155] Darbre PD, Aljarrah A, Miller WR, Coldham NG, Sauer MJ, Pope GS. Concentrations of parabens in human breast tumours. *J Appl Toxicol. 2004Jan-Feb;24(1):5-13.*

[156] Crinnion WJ. Toxic effects of the easily avoidable phthalates and parabens. *Altern Med Rev. 2010 Sep;15(3):190-6.*

[157] Zitting A, Heinonen T. Decrease of reduced glutathione in isolated rat hepatocytes caused by acrolein, acrylonitrile, and the thermal degradation products of styrene copolymers. *Toxicology. 1980;17(3):333-41.*

[158] Centers for Disease Control and Prevention (CDC). Illnesses associated with occupational use of flea-control products--California, Texas, and Washington, 1989-1997. *MMWR Morb Mortal Wkly Rep. 1999 Jun 4;48(21):443-7.*

[159] de la Cerda E, Navarro-Polanco RA, Sánchez-Chapula JA. Modulation of cardiac action potential and underlying ionic currents by the pyrethroid insecticide deltamethrin. *Arch Med Res. 2002 Sep-Oct;33(5):448-54.*

[160] Abdel-Khalik MM, Hanafy MS, Abdel-Aziz MI. Studies on the teratogenic effects of deltamethrin in rats. *Dtsch Tierarztl Wochenschr. 1993 Apr;100(4):142-3.*

[161] Pagès N, Sauviat MP, Bouvet S, Goudey-Perrière F. Reproductive toxicity of lindane. *J Soc Biol. 2002;196(4):325-38.*

[162] Ward MH, Colt JS, Metayer C, Gunier RB, Lubin J, Crouse V, Nishioka MG, Reynolds P, Buffler PA. Residential exposure to polychlorinated biphenyls and organochlorine pesticides and risk of childhood leukemia. *Environ Health Perspect. 2009 Jun;117(6):1007-13.*

[163] Chen J, Schenker S, Henderson GI. 4-hydroxynonenal detoxification by mitochondrial glutathione S-transferase is compromised by short-term ethanol consumption in rats. *Alcohol Clin Exp Res. 2002 Aug;26(8):1252-8.*

[164] Tielemans E, Heederik D, Burdorf A, Vermeulen R, Veulemans H, Kromhout H,Hartog K. Assessment of occupational exposures in a general population: comparison of different methods. *Occup Environ Med. 1999 Mar;56(3):145-51.*

[165] Wagner U, Schlebusch H, van der Ven H, van der Ven K, Diedrich K, Krebs D. Accumulation of pollutants in the genital tract of sterility patients. *J Clin Chem Clin Biochem. 1990 Oct;28(10):683-8.*

[166] Cicero TJ, Nock B, O'Connor L, Adams ML, Sewing BN, Meyer ER. Acute alcohol exposure markedly influences male fertility and fetal outcome in the male rat. *Life Sci. 1994;55(12):901-10.*

[167] Hadi HA, Hill JA, Castillo RA. Alcohol and reproductive function: a review. *Obstet Gynecol Surv. 1987 Feb;42(2):69-74.*

[168] Aschengrau A, Weinberg JM, Janulewicz PA, Romano ME, Gallagher LG, Winter MR, Martin BR, Vieira VM, Webster TF, White RF, Ozonoff DM. Affinity for risky behaviors following prenatal and early childhood exposure to tetrachloroethylene(PCE)-contaminated drinking water: a retrospective cohort study. *Environ Health. 2011 Dec 2;10:102.*

[169] Epstein SS, Ozonoff D. Leukemias and blood dyscrasias following exposure to chlordane and heptachlor. *Teratog Carcinog Mutagen. 1987;7(6):527-40.*

[170] Allen RH, Gottlieb M, Clute E, Pongsiri MJ, Sherman J, Obrams GI. Breast cancer and pesticides in Hawaii: the need for further study. *Environ Health Perspect. 1997 Apr;105 Suppl 3:679-83.*

[171] Trocho C, Pardo R, Rafecas I, Virgili J, Remesar X, Fernández-López JA, Alemany M. Formaldehyde derived from dietary aspartame binds to tissue components in vivo. *Life Sci. 1998;63(5):337-49.*

[172] Seltzer JM. Biologic contaminants. *Occup Med. 1995 Jan-Mar;10(1):1-25.*

[173] Fasano A, Shea-Donohue T. Mechanisms of disease: the role of intestinal barrier function in the pathogenesis of gastrointestinal autoimmune diseases. *Nat Clin Pract Gastroenterol Hepatol. 2005 Sep;2(9):416-22.*

[174] Maia-Brigagão C, Morgado-Díaz JA, De Souza W. Giardia disrupts the arrangement of tight, adherens and desmosomal junction proteins of intestinal cells. *Parasitol Int. 2012 Jun;61(2):280-7.*

[175] Lejeune M, Moreau F, Chadee K. Prostaglandin E2 produced by Entamoeba histolytica signals via EP4 receptor and alters claudin-4 to increase ion permeability of tight junctions. *Am J Pathol. 2011 Aug;179(2):807-18.*

[176] Bjarnason I, Peters TJ, Wise RJ. The leaky gut of alcoholism: possible route of entry for toxic compounds. *Lancet. 1984 Jan 28;1(8370):179-82.*

[177] Maes M, Kubera M, Leunis JC. The gut-brain barrier in major depression: intestinal mucosal dysfunction with an increased translocation of LPS from gram negative enterobacteria (leaky gut) plays a role in the inflammatory pathophysiology of depression. *Neuro Endocrinol Lett. 2008 Feb;29(1):117-24.*

[178] Su CW, Cao Y, Kaplan J, Zhang M, Li W, Conroy M, Walker WA, Shi HN. Duodenal helminth infection alters barrier function of the colonic epithelium via adaptive immune activation. *Infect Immun. 2011 Jun;79(6):2285-94.*

[179] Lloyd DJ, Helmering J, Cordover D, Bowsman M, Chen M, Hale C, Fordstrom P,Zhou M, Wang M, Kaufman SA, Véniant MM. Antidiabetic effects of 11beta-HSD1 inhibition in a mouse model of combined diabetes, dyslipidaemia and atherosclerosis. *Diabetes Obes Metab. 2009 Jul;11(7):688-99.*

[180] Deslypere JP, Verdonck L, Vermeulen A. Fat tissue: a steroid reservoir and site of steroid metabolism. *J Clin Endocrinol Metab. 1985 Sep;61(3):564-70.*

[181] Ukkola O, Santaniemi M. Adiponectin: a link between excess adiposity and associated comorbidities? *J Mol Med (Berl). 2002 Nov;80(11):696-702.*

[182] Yang Q, Graham TE, Mody N, Preitner F, Peroni OD, Zabolotny JM, Kotani K, Quadro L, Kahn BB (2005). "Serum retinol binding protein 4 contributes to insulin resistance in obesity and type 2 diabetes". *Nature 436 (7049): 356–62.*

[183] Epel E, Lapidus R, McEwen B, Brownell K. Stress may add bite to appetite in women: a laboratory study of stress-induced cortisol and eating behavior. *Psychoneuroendocrinology 2001 Jan;26(1):37-49*

[184] Cavagnini F, Croci M. Putignano P., et al. Glucocorticoids and neuroendocrine function. *International Journal of Obesity 24:577-579, 2000.*

[185] Hoffman SW, Virmani S, Simkins RM, Stein DG. The delayed administration of dehydroepiandrosterone sulfate improves recovery of function after traumatic brain injury in rats. *J Neurotrauma. 2003 Sep;20(9):859-70.*

[186] Rosero-Bixby L, Dow WH. Predicting mortality with biomarkers: a population-based prospective cohort study for elderly Costa Ricans. *Popul Health Metr. 2012 Jun 13;10(1):11.*

[187] Weiss EP, Villareal DT, Ehsani AA, Fontana L, Holloszy JO. Dehydroepiandrosterone replacement therapy in older adults improves indices of arterial stiffness. *Aging Cell. 2012 Jun 19.*

[188] Knudsen N, Laurberg P, Rasmussen LB, Bülow I, Perrild H, Ovesen L, Jørgensen T. Small differences in thyroid function may be important for body mass index and the occurrence of obesity in the population. *J Clin Endocrinol Metab. 2005 Jul;90(7):4019-24.*

[189] Attie AD, Scherer PE. Adipocyte metabolism and obesity. *J Lipid Res. 2009 Apr;50 Suppl:S395-9.*

[190] Hotta M, Ohwada R, Akamizu T, Shibasaki T, Takano K, Kangawa K. Ghrelin increases hunger and food intake in patients with restricting-type anorexia nervosa: a pilot study. *Endocr J. 2009;56(9):1119-28.*

[191] Zhang N, Yuan C, Li Z, Li J, Li X, Li C, Li R, Wang SR. Meta-analysis of the relationship between obestatin and ghrelin levels and the ghrelin/obestatin ratio with respect to obesity. *Am J Med Sci. 2011 Jan;341(1):48-55.*

[192] Mullerova D, Kopecky J, Matejkova D, et al. Negative association between plasma levels of adiponectin and polychlorinated biphenyl 153 in obese women under non-energy-restrictive regime. *Int J Obes (Lond). Dec 2008;32(12):1875-1878.*

[193] Lee J, Hopkins V. *What Your Doctor May Not Tell You About Menopause.* New York, New York: Warner Books, 1996.

[194] Korenman SG, Morley JE, Mooradian AD, Davis SS, Kaiser FE, Silver AJ, Viosca SP, Garza D. Secondary hypogonadism in older men: its relation to impotence. *J Clin Endocrinol Metab. 1990 Oct;71(4):963-9.*

[195] Fuhrman BJ, Schairer C, Gail MH, Boyd-Morin J, Xu X, Sue LY, Buys SS, Isaacs C, Keefer LK, Veenstra TD, Berg CD, Hoover RN, Ziegler RG. Estrogen metabolism and risk of breast cancer in postmenopausal women. *J Natl Cancer Inst. 2012 Feb 22;104(4):326-39.*

[196] Napoli N, Vattikuti S, Yarramaneni J, Giri TK, Nekkalapu S, Qualls C, Armamento-Villareal RC. Increased 2-hydroxylation of estrogen is associated with lower body fat and increased lean body mass in postmenopausal women. *Maturitas. 2012 Feb 29.*

[197] Castagnetta LA, Granata OM, Traina A, Ravazzolo B, Amoroso M, Miele M, Bellavia V, Agostara B, Carruba G. Tissue content of hydroxyestrogens in relation to survival of breast cancer patients. *Clin Cancer Res. 2002 Oct;8(10):3146-55.*

[198] Yager JD, Liehr JG. Molecular mechanisms of estrogen carcinogenesis. *Annu Rev Pharmacol Toxicol. 1996;36:203-32.*

[199] Wright YL. *Secrets about Bioidentical Hormones to Lose Fat and Prevent Cancer, Heart Disease, Menopause, and Andropause, by Optimizing Adrenals, Thyroid, Estrogen, Progesterone, Testosterone, and Growth Hormone!* Lulu.com. 2010.

[200] Hayes CL, Spink DC, Spink BC, Cao JQ, Walker NJ, Sutter TR. 17 beta-estradiol hydroxylation catalyzed by human cytochrome P450 1B1. *Proc Natl Acad Sci U S A. 1996 Sep 3;93(18):9776-81.*

[201] Kugaya A, Epperson CN, Zoghbi S, van Dyck CH, Hou Y, Fujita M, Staley JK, Garg PK, Seibyl JP, Innis RB. Increase in prefrontal cortex serotonin 2A receptors following estrogen treatment in postmenopausal women. *Am J Psychiatry. 2003 Aug;160(8):1522-4.*

[202] Fink G, Sumner BE, Rosie R, Grace O, Quinn JP. Estrogen control of central neurotransmission: effect on mood, mental state, and memory. *Cell Mol Neurobiol. 1996 Jun;16(3):325-44.*

[203] Crinnion WJ. The benefits of pre- and post-challenge urine heavy metal testing: Part 1. *Altern Med Rev. 2009 Mar;14(1):3-8.*

[204] Crinnion WJ. Chlorinated pesticides: threats to health and importance of detection. *Altern Med Rev. 2009 Dec;14(4):347-59.*

[205] Crinnion WJ. The role of persistent organic pollutants in the worldwide epidemic of type 2 diabetes mellitus and the possible connection to Farmed Atlantic Salmon (Salmo salar). *Altern Med Rev. 2011 Dec;16(4):301-13.*

[206] Hartle R. Exposure to methyl tert-butyl ether and benzene among service station attendants and operators. *Environ Health Perspect. 1993 Dec;101 Suppl 6:23-6.*

[207] O'Keefe JH, Gheewala NM, O'Keefe JO. Dietary strategies for improving post-prandial glucose, lipids, inflammation, and cardiovascular health. *J Am Coll Cardiol. 2008 Jan 22;51(3):249-55.*

[208] Clemmons, DR. Commercial assays available for insulin-like growth factor I and their use in diagnosing growth hormone deficiency. *Horm Res. 2001; 55 Suppl 2:73-9.*

[209] Muti P, Bradlow HL, Micheli A, Krogh V, Freudenheim JL, Schünemann HJ, Stanulla M, Yang J, Sepkovic DW, Trevisan M, Berrino F. Estrogen metabolism and risk of breast cancer: a prospective study of the 2:16 alpha-hydroxyestrone ratio in premenopausal and postmenopausal women. *Epidemiology. 2000 Nov;11(6):635-40.*

[210] Anand P, Kunnumakkara AB, Sundaram C, Harikumar KB, Tharakan ST, Lai OS, Sung B, Aggarwal BB. Cancer is a preventable disease that requires major lifestyle changes. *Pharm Res. 2008 Sep;25(9):2097-116.*

[211] Lietava J, B BV, Dukat A, Fodor GJ. Homocysteine Slovakia study: study design and occurrence of hyperhomocysteinaemia and other risk factors. *Bratisl Lek Listy. 2012;113(2):80-6.*

[212] Song IU, Kim YD, Kim JS, Lee KS, Chung SW. Can high-sensitivity C-reactive protein and plasma homocysteine levels independently predict the prognosis of patients with functional disability after first-ever ischemic stroke? *Eur Neurol. 010;64(5):304-10.*

[213] Agnati LF, Genedani S, Leo G, Forni A, Woods AS, Filaferro M, Franco R, Fuxe K. Abeta peptides as one of the crucial volume transmission signals in the trophic units and their interactions with homocysteine. Physiological implications and relevance for Alzheimer's disease. *J Neural Transm. 2007 Jan;114(1):21-31.*

[214] Bucciarelli P, Martini G, Martinelli I, Ceccarelli E, Gennari L, Bader R, Valenti R, Franci B, Nuti R, Mannucci PM. The relationship between plasma homocysteine levels and bone mineral density in post-menopausal women. *Eur J Intern Med. 2010 Aug;21(4):301-5.*

[215] Peto MV. Aluminium and iron in humans: bioaccumulation, pathology, and removal. *Rejuvenation Res. 2010 Oct;13(5):589-98.*

[216] Ferriby LL, Knutsen JS, Harris M, et al. Evaluation of PCDD/F and dioxin-like PCB serum concentration data from the 2001-2002 National Health and Nutrition Examination Survey of the United States population. *J Expo Sci Environ Epidemiol. Jul 2007;17(4):358-371.*

[217] Walker P, Rhubart-Berg P, McKenzie S, Kelling K, Lawrence RS. Public health implications of meat production and consumption. *Public Health Nutr. Jun 2005;8(4):348-356.*

[218] Dagnelie PC, van Staveren WA, Roos AH, Tuinstra LG, Burema J. Nutrients and contaminants in human milk from mothers on macrobiotic and omnivorous diets. *Eur J Clin Nutr. May 1992;46(5):355-366.*

[219] Craig WJ, Mangels AR. Position of the American Dietetic Association: vegetarian diets. *J Am Diet Assoc. Jul 2009;109(7):1266-1282.*

[220] García-Prieto A, Lunar L, Rubio S, Pérez-Bendito D. Decanoic acid reverse micelle-based coacervates for the microextraction of bisphenol A from canned vegetables and fruits. *Anal Chim Acta. 2008 Jun 9;617(1-2):51-8.*

[221] Cao XL, Corriveau J, Popovic S. Sources of low concentrations of bisphenol A in canned beverage products. *J Food Prot. 2010 Aug;73(8):1548-51.*

[222] Ferrucci LM, Sinha R, Ward MH, Graubard BI, Hollenbeck AR, Kilfoy BA, Schatzkin A, Michaud DS, Cross AJ. Meat and components of meat and the risk of bladder cancer in the NIH-AARP Diet and Health Study. *Cancer. 2010 Sep 15;116(18):4345-53.*

[223] Alexander JC. Chemical and biological properties related to toxicity of heated fats. *J Toxicol Environ Health. 1981 Jan;7(1):125-38.*

[224] Castro-Martínez MG, Bolado-García VE, Landa-Anell MV, Liceaga-Cravioto MG,Soto-González J, López-Alvarenga JC. Dietary trans fatty acids and its metabolic implications. *Gac Med Mex. 2010 Jul-Aug;146(4):281-8.*

[225] Crinnion WJ. Organic foods contain higher levels of certain nutrients, lower levels of pesticides, and may provide health benefits for the consumer. *Altern Med Rev. 2010 Apr;15(1):4-12.*

[226] Kulvinskas, V. *Survival into the 21st Century.* Omangod Press. 1975.

[227] http://www.ewg.org/foodnews/summary/

[228] Cummings SR, Tripp MK, Herrmann NB. Approaches to the prevention and control of skin cancer. *Cancer Metastasis Rev. 1997 Sep-Dec;16(3-4):309-27.*

[229] Wolf P, Donawho CK, Kripke ML. Effect of sunscreens on UV radiation-induced enhancement of melanoma growth in mice. *J Natl Cancer Inst. 1994 Jan 19;86(2):99-105.*

[230] James SJ, Slikker W 3rd, Melnyk S, New E, Pogribna M, Jernigan S. Thimerosal neurotoxicity is associated with glutathione depletion: protection with glutathione precursors. *Neurotoxicology. 2005 Jan;26(1):1-8.*

[231] Donpunha W, Kukongviriyapan U, Sompamit K, Pakdeechote P, Kukongviriyapan V, Pannangpetch P. Protective effect of ascorbic acid on cadmium-induced hypertension and vascular dysfunction in mice. *Biometals. 2011 Feb;24(1):105-15.*

[232] Ros E, Tapsell LC, Sabaté J. Nuts and berries for heart health. *Curr Atheroscler Rep. 2010 Nov;12(6):397-406.*

[233] Weaver CM, Martin BR, Story JA, Hutchinson I, Sanders L. Novel Fibers Increase Bone Calcium Content and Strength beyond Efficiency of Large Intestine Fermentation. *J Agric Food Chem. 2010 Aug 2.*

[234] Bidoli E, Pelucchi C, Zucchetto A, Negri E, Dal Maso L, Polesel J, Montella M, Franceschi S, Serraino D, La Vecchia C, Talamini R. Fiber intake and endometrial cancer risk. *Acta Oncol. 2010 May;49(4):441-6.*

[235] Thieu NQ, Ogle B, Pettersson H. Efficacy of bentonite clay in ameliorating aflatoxicosis in piglets fed aflatoxin contaminated diets. *Trop Anim Health Prod.2008 Dec;40(8):649-56.*

[236] Fork FT, Ekberg O, Nilsson G, Rerup C, Skinhøj A. Colon cleansing regimens. A clinical study in 1200 patients. *Gastrointest Radiol. 1982;7(4):383-9.*

[237] Gerson M. The cure of advanced cancer by diet therapy: a summary of 30 years of clinical experimentation. *Physiol Chem Phys. 1978;10(5):449-64.*

238 Lam LK, Sparnins VL, Wattenberg LW. Effects of derivatives of kahweol and cafestol on the activity of glutathione S-transferase in mice. *J Med Chem. 1987 Aug;30(8):1399-403.*

239 Uchikawa T, Yasutake A, Kumamoto Y, Maruyama I, Kumamoto S, Ando Y. The influence of Parachlorella beyerinckii CK-5 on the absorption and excretion of methylmercury (MeHg) in mice. *J Toxicol Sci. 2010;35(1):101-5.*

240 Pore RS. Detoxification of chlordecone poisoned rats with chlorella and chlorella derived sporopollenin. *Drug Chem Toxicol. 1984;7(1):57-71.*

241 Huang Z, Li L, Huang G, Yan Q, Shi B, Xu X. Growth-inhibitory and metal-binding proteins in Chlorella vulgaris exposed to cadmium or zinc. *Aquat Toxicol. 2009 Jan 18;91(1):54-61.*

242 Feldman DN, Feldman JG, Greenblatt R, Anastos K, Pearce L, Cohen M, Gange S, Leanza S, Burk R. CYP1A1 genotype modifies the impact of smoking on effectiveness of HAART among women. *AIDS Educ Prev. 2009 Jun;21(3 Suppl):81-93.*

243 Rothman N, Shields PG, Poirier MC, Harrington AM, Ford DP, Strickland PT. The impact of glutathione s-transferase M1 and cytochrome P450 1A1 genotypes on white-blood-cell polycyclic aromatic hydrocarbon-DNA adduct levels in humans. *Mol Carcinog. 1995 Sep;14(1):63-8.*

244 Kovacic P, Somanathan R. Dermal toxicity and environmental contamination: electron transfer, reactive oxygen species, oxidative stress, cell signaling, and protection by antioxidants. *Rev Environ Contam Toxicol. 2010;203:119-38.*

245 Epstein HA. Food for thought and skin. *Skinmed. 2010 Jan-Feb;8(1):50-1.*

246 Franco JL, Posser T, Missau F, Pizzolatti MG, Dos Santos AR, Souza DO, Aschner M, Rocha JB, Dafre AL, Farina M. Structure-activity relationship of flavonoids derived from medicinal plants in preventing methylmercury-induced mitochondrial dysfunction. *Environ Toxicol Pharmacol. 2010 Nov 1;30(3):272-278.*

247 Genuis SJ, Birkholz D, Ralitsch M, Thibault N. Human detoxification of perfluorinated compounds. *Public Health. 2010 Jul;124(7):367-75.*

248 Krop J. Chemical sensitivity after intoxication at work with solvents: response to sauna therapy. *J Altern Complement Med. 1998 Spring;4(1):77-86.*

249 Sobajima M, Nozawa T, Ihori H, Shida T, Ohori T, Suzuki T, Matsuki A, Yasumura S, Inoue H. Repeated sauna therapy improves myocardial perfusion in patients with chronically occluded coronary artery-related ischemia. *Int J Cardiol. 2012 Jan 12.*

250 Hsu YH, Chen YC, Chen TH, Sue YM, Cheng TH, Chen JR, Chen CH. Far-infrared therapy induces the nuclear translocation of PLZF which inhibits VEGF-induced proliferation in human umbilical vein endothelial cells. *PLoS One.2012;7(1):e30674.*

251 Wong CH, Lin LC, Lee HH, Liu CF. The analgesic effect of thermal therapy after total knee arthroplasty. *J Altern Complement Med. 2012 Feb;18(2):175-9.*

252 Chang Y, Liu YP, Liu CF. The effect on serotonin and MDA levels in depressed patients with insomnia when far-infrared rays are applied to acupoints. *Am J Chin Med. 2009;37(5):837-42.*

253 Matsushita K, Masuda A, Tei C. Efficacy of Waon therapy for fibromyalgia. *Intern Med. 2008;47(16):1473-6.*

254 Beever R. Far-infrared saunas for treatment of cardiovascular risk factors: summary of published evidence. *Can Fam Physician. 2009 Jul;55(7):691-6.*

255 Crinnion WJ. Sauna as a valuable clinical tool for cardiovascular, autoimmune, toxicant- induced and other chronic health problems. *Altern Med Rev. 2011 Sep;16(3):215-25.*

256 Masuda A, Kihara T, Fukudome T, Shinsato T, Minagoe S, Tei C. The effects of repeated thermal therapy for two patients with chronic fatigue syndrome. *J Psychosom Res. 2005 Apr;58(4):383-7.*

257 Bloomer RJ, Kabir MM, Canale RE, Trepanowski JF, Marshall KE, Farney TM, Hammond KG. Effect of a 21 day Daniel Fast on metabolic and cardiovascular disease risk factors in men and women. *Lipids Health Dis. 2010 Sep 3;9:94.*

258 Crinnion WJ. The benefit of pre- and post-challenge urine heavy metal testing: part 2. *Altern Med Rev. 2009 Jun;14(2):103-8.*

259 Machida M, Sun SJ, Oguma E, Kayama F. High bone matrix turnover predicts blood levels of lead among perimenopausal women. *Environ Res. 2009 Oct;109(7):880-6.*

260 See D, Mason S, Roshan R. Increased tumor necrosis factor alpha (TNF-alpha) and natural killer cell (NK) function using an integrative approach in late stage cancers. *Immunol Invest. 2002 May;31(2):137-53.*

261 Sergeev, AV. Correction of biochemical and immunological indices in colonic cancer using optimal doses of retinyl acetate and ascorbic acid. *Biull Eksp Biol Med. 1983 Sep;96(9):90-2.*

262 el-Adhami W, Daly S, Stewart PR. Biochemical studies on the lethal effects of solar and artificial ultraviolet radiation on Staphylococcus aureus. *Arch Microbiol. 1994;161(1):82-7.*

263 Ukena SN, Singh A, Dringenberg U, Engelhardt R, Seidler U, Hansen W, Bleich A, Bruder D, Franzke A, Rogler G, Suerbaum S, Buer J, Gunzer F, Westendorf AM. Probiotic Escherichia coli Nissle 1917 inhibits leaky gut by

enhancing mucosal integrity. *PLoS One. 2007 Dec 12;2(12):e1308.*

[264] Hollander D. Intestinal permeability, leaky gut, and intestinal disorders. *Curr Gastroenterol Rep. 1999 Oct;1(5):410-6.*

[265] Gorbach SL. Goldin BR. Nutrition and the gastrointestinal microflora. *Nutr Rev 1992; 50:378-381.*

[266] Keller JB, Bevier WC, Jovanovic-Peterson L, Formby B, Durak EP, Peterson CM. Voluntary exercise improves glycemia in non-obese diabetic (NOD) mice. *Diabetes Res Clin Pract. 1993 Oct-Nov;22(1):29-35.*

[267] Cleare AJ, Miell J, Heap E, Sookdeo S, Young L, Malhi GS, O'Keane V. Hypothalamo-pituitary-adrenal axis dysfunction in chronic fatigue syndrome, and the effects of low-dose hydrocortisone therapy. *J Clin Endocrinol Metab. 2001 Aug;86(8):3545-54.*

[268] Langer P. The impacts of organochlorines and other persistent pollutants on thyroid and metabolic health. *Front Neuroendocrinol. 2010 Oct;31(4):497-518.*

[269] Wright YL, *Secrets about Bioidentical Hormones to Lose Fat and Prevent Cancer, Heart Disease, Menopause, and Andropause, by Optimizing Adrenals, Thyroid, Estrogen, Progesterone, Testosterone, and Growth Hormone!* Lulu.com. 2010. p 30.

[270] Wright YL. *Bioidentical Hormones Made Easy!* Lulu.com. 2011. p34.

[271] Devlin A. et al., "Hyperhomocysteinemia," in Glew, T., and Rosenthal, M., ed., *3rd* ed. New York: Oxford University Press, 2007, *Clinical Studies in Medical Biochemistry,* p 226-233.

[272] Heerdt AS, Young CW, Borgen PI. Calcium glucarate as a chemopreventive agent in breast cancer. *Altern Med Rev. 2002 Aug; 7(4):336-9.*

[273] Decensi A, Omodei U, Robertson C, Bonanni B, Guerrieri-Gonzaga A, Ramazzotto F, Johansson H, Mora S, Sandri MT, Cazzaniga M, Franchi M, Pecorelli S. Effect of transdermal estradiol and oral conjugated estrogen on C-reactive protein in retinoid-placebo trial in healthy women. *Circulation 2002 Sep 3;106(10):1224-8.*

[274] Notelovitz M. Androgen effects on bone and muscle. *Fertil Steril. 2002 Apr;77 Suppl 4:S34-41.*

[275] Roddam AW, Allen NE, Appleby P, Key TJ. Endogenous Hormones and Prostate Cancer Collaborative Group. Endogenous Sex Hormones and Prostate Cancer: A Collaborative Analysis of 18 Prospective Studies. *J Natl Cancer Inst. 2008 Feb 6;100(3):170-83.*

[276] Gould DC. and Kirby RS. Testosterone replacement therapy for late onset hypogonadism: what is the risk of inducing prostate cancer? *Prostate Cancer Prostatic Dis. 2006; 9(1):14-8.*

[277] Feneley MR, Carruthers ME. PSA monitoring during testosterone replacement therapy: low long-term risk of prostate cancer with improved opportunity for cure. *Andrologia 2004; 36:212.*

[278] Marks LS, Mazer NA, Mostaghel E, Hess DL, Dorey FJ, Epstein JI, Veltri RW, Makarov DV, Partin AW, Bostwick DG, Macairan ML, Nelson PS. Effect of testosterone replacement therapy on prostate tissue in men with late-onset hypogonadism: a randomized controlled trial. *JAMA. 2006 Nov 15;296(19):2351-61.*

[279] Wright YL, *Secrets about Bioidentical Hormones to Lose Fat and Prevent Cancer, Heart Disease, Menopause, and Andropause, by Optimizing Adrenals, Thyroid, Estrogen, Progesterone, Testosterone, and Growth Hormone!* Lulu.com. 2010. p 35.

[280] Malkin CJ, Pugh PJ, Jones RD, Kapoor D, Channer KS, Jones TH. The effect of testosterone replacement on endogenous inflammatory cytokines and lipid profiles in hypogonadal men. *J Clin Endocrinol Metab. 2004 Jul;89(7):33118-8.*

[281] Channer KS, Jones TH. Cardiovascular effects of testosterone: implications of the "male menopause"? *Heart. 2003 Feb;89(2):121-2.*

[282] English KM, Steeds RP, Jones TH, Diver MJ, Channer KS. Low-dose transdermal testosterone therapy improves angina threshold in men with chronic stable angina: A randomized, double-blind, placebo-controlled study. *Circulation 2000. Oct 17; 102(16):1906-11.*

[283] Malkin CJ, Pugh PJ, Morris PD, Kerry KE, Jones RD, Jones TH, Channer KS. Testosterone replacement in hypogonadal men with angina improves ischaemic threshold and quality of life. *Heart. 2004 Aug;90(8):871-6.*

[284] Rosano GM, Leonardo F, Pagnotta P, Pelliccia F, Panina G, Cerquetani E, della Monica PL, Bonfigli B, Volpe M, Chierchia SL. Acute anti-ischemic effect of testosterone in men with coronary artery disease. *Circulation 1999 Apr 6;99(13):1666-70.*

[285] Webb CM, McNeill JG, Hayward CS, de Zeigler D, Collins P. Effects of testosterone on coronary vasomotor regulation in men with coronary heart disease. *Circulation. 1999 Oct 19;100(16):1690-6.*

[286] Khaw KT, Barrett-Connor E. Blood pressure and endogenous testosterone in men: an inverse relationship. *J Hypertens. 1988 Apr;6(4):329-32.*

[287] Bhasin S. The dose-dependent effects of testosterone on sexual function and on muscle mass and function. *Mayo Clin Proc. 2000 Jan;75 Suppl:S70-5.*

[288] Boyanov MA, Boneva Z, Christov VG. Testosterone supplementation in men with type 2 diabetes, visceral obesity and partial androgen deficiency. *Aging Male. 2003 Mar; 6(1):1-7.*

[289] Cooper MA, Ritchie EC. Testosterone replacement therapy for anxiety. *Am J Psychiatry. 2000 Nov;157(11):1884.*

[290] Alexander GM, Swerdloff RS, Wang C, Davidson T, McDonald V, Steiner B, Hines M. Androgen-behavior correlations in hypogonadal men and eugonadal men. *II. Cognitive abilities. Horm Behav. 1998 Apr;33(2):85-94.*

[291] Barrett-Connor E, Goodman-Gruen D, Patay B. Endogenous sex hormones and cognitive function in older men. *J Clin Endocrinol Metab 1999 Oct; 84(10):3681-5.*

[292] Moffat SD, Resnick SM. Long-term measures of free testosterone predict regional cerebral blood flow patterns in elderly men. *Neurobiol Aging. 2007 Jun;28(6):914-20.*

[293] Gouras GK, Xu H, Gross RS, Greenfield JP, Hai B, Wang R, Greengard P. Testosterone reduces neuronal secretion of beta amyloid peptides. *Proc Natl Acad Sci U S A 2000 Feb 1;97(3):1202-5.*

[294] Tan RS, Pu SJ. A pilot study on the effects of testosterone in hypogonadal aging male patients with Alzheimer's disease. *Aging Male. 3003 Mar;6(1):13-7.*

[295] Burris AS, Banks SM, Carter CS, Davidson JM, Sherins RJ. A long-term, prospective study of the physiologic and behavioral effects of hormone replacement in untreated hypogonadal men. *J Androl 1992 Jul-Aug; 13(4)297-304.*

[296] Caretta N, Ferlin A, Palego PF, Foresta C. Erectile dysfunction in aging men: testosterone role in therapeutic protocols. *J Endocrinol Invest. 2005;28(11 Suppl Proceedings):108-11.*

[297] Foresta C, Caretta N, Lana A, De Toni L, Biagioli A, Ferlin A, Garolla A. Reduced number of circulating Endothelial Progenitor Cells in hypogonadal men. *Journal of Clinical Endocrinology and Metabolism 91(11)4599-4602.*

[298] Muniyappa R, Sorkin JD, Veldhuis JD, Harman SM, Münzer T, Bhasin S, Blackman MR. Long-term testosterone supplementation augments overnight growth hormone secretion in healthy older men. *Am J Physiol Endocrinol Metab. 2007 Sep;293(3):E769-75.*

[299] Leder BZ, Rohrer JL, Rubin SD, Gallo J, Longcope C. Effects of aromatase inhibition in elderly men with low or borderline-low serum testosterone levels. *J Clin Endocrinol Metab. 2004 Mar;89(3):1174-80.*

[300] Jeong HJ, Shin YG, Kim IH, Pezzuto JM. Inhibition of aromatase activity by flavonoids. *Arch Pharm Res. 1999 Jun:22(3):309-12.*

[301] Malaab SA, Pollak MN, Goodyer CG. Direct effects of tamoxifen on growth hormone secretion by pituitary cells in vitro. *Eur J Cancer. 1992;28A(4-5):788-93.*

[302] Bradlow HL, Telang NT, Sepkovic DW, Osborne MP. 2-hydroxyestrone: the 'good' estrogen. *J Endocrinol. 1996 Sep;150 Suppl:S259-65.*

[303] Fishman J, Schneider J, Hershcope RJ, Bradlow HL. Increased estrogen-16 alpha-hydroxylase activity in women with breast and endometrial cancer. *J Steroid Biochem. 1984 Apr;20(4B):1077-81.*

[304] Muti P, Bradlow HL, Micheli A, Krogh V, Freudenheim JL, Schünemann HJ, Stanulla M, Yang J, Sepkovic DW, Trevisan M, Berrino F. Estrogen metabolism and risk of breast cancer: a prospective study of the 2:16 alpha-hydroxyestrone ratio in premenopausal and postmenopausal women. *Epidemiology. 2000 Nov;11(6):635-40.*

[305] Liehr JG, Ricci MJ. 4-Hydroxylation of estrogens as marker of human mammary tumors. *Proc Natl Acad Sci U S A. 1996 Apr 16;93(8):3294-6.*

[306] Sepkovic DW, Stein J, Carlisle AD, Ksieski HB, Auborn K, Bradlow HL. Diindolylmethane inhibits cervical dysplasia, alters estrogen metabolism, and enhances immune response in the K14-HPV16 transgenic mouse model. *Cancer Epidemiol Biomarkers Prev. 2009 Nov;18(11):2957-64.*

[307] Hsu PC, Guo YL. Antioxidant nutrients and lead toxicity. *Toxicology. 2002 Oct 30;180(1):33-44.*

[308] Beasley CL, Honer WG, Bergmann K, Falkai P, Lütjohann D, Bayer TA. Reductions in cholesterol and synaptic markers in association cortex in mood disorders. *Bipolar Disord. 2005 Oct;7(5):449-55.*

[309] Landmark K, Reikvam A. [Nutrition, dietary supplementation and coronary heart disease]. *Tidsskr Nor Laegeforen. 2000 Sep 20;120(22):2648-53.*

[310] Klaiber EL, Broverman DM, Vogel W, Peterson LG, Snyder MB. Individual differences in changes in mood and platelet monoamine oxidase (MAO) activity during hormonal replacement therapy in menopausal women. *Psychoneuroendocrinology. 1996 Oct;21(7):575-92.*

[311] Pluchino N, Lenzi E, Merlini S, Giannini A, Cubeddu A, Casarosa E, Begliuomini S, Luisi M, Cela V, Genazzani AR. Progesterone and progestins: effects on brain, allopregnenolone and beta-endorphin. *J Steroid Biochem Mol Biol. 2006.*

INDEX

5-alpha reductase, 71
acetylcholine, 32, 76
acne, 28, 30, 31
adaptogens, 64, 65, 66
addiction, 32
adrenal, 26, 27, 28, 30, 31, 40, 54, 64, 65, 66
alcohol, 32, 47, 61, 66, 75, 77
allergies, 24, 30
Alzheimer's, 31, 68, 70, 76
anastrozole, 69
androgens, 69, 70
andropause, 28
antibiotics, 11, 22, 23, 40, 45, 58, 59, 61
antidepressants, 28, 69, 70, 75
antioxidants, 51, 62, 63
anxiety, 27, 32, 64, 66, 75, 77
appetite, 8, 25, 27, 29
aromatases, 31, 71
arthritis, 9, 53, 70
autoimmunity, 28, 41, 72
BHRT, 34, 41, 67, 76
binging, 32, 76
bioidentical, 65, 67, 68, 69, 76
bladder, 50, 57, 61
blood clots, 69
blood pressure, 26, 64, 65, 68, 69, 70
blood sugar, 26, 27, 28, 30, 35, 41, 54, 63
bone, 30, 31, 68, 69, 71
breast cancer, 12, 14, 17, 18, 20, 28, 30, 53, 67, 68, 71
breast tenderness, 67
caffeine, 47, 64, 76
Calcium D-Glucarate, 52, 68
cancer, 11, 12, 14, 15, 28, 30, 49, 50, 51, 57, 58, 61, 63, 67, 68, 69, 70, 72, 74
carbohydrate, 27, 28, 61, 63, 64, 75, 76
cardiovascular, 30, 64, 69, 71, 72
chelation, 55
cholesterol, 64, 70, 74
coffee enemas, 50
colonics, 49
Cortef, 64, 65, 66
cortisol, 26, 27, 28, 30, 34, 40, 64, 65, 66
cravings, 27, 28, 32, 75
C-reactive protein, 35, 69

depression, 29, 31, 32, 75
DHEA, 27, 28, 31, 35, 42, 63, 64, 66, 76
DHT, 71
diabetes, 6, 7, 15, 16, 41, 50, 62
diet, 11, 29, 30, 32, 47, 57, 61, 63, 64, 66, 67, 68, 69, 75
digestion, 34, 38, 60
dioxin, 20, 21, 37, 53
dopamine, 32, 65, 76
dysbiosis, 11, 22, 23, 24, 25, 38, 39, 57, 59, 61
enemas, 49, 50, 54, 61
enzymes, 28, 29, 31, 61, 63, 71
erectile dysfunction, 35, 42, 70
estradiol, 30, 41, 71
estrogen, 26, 29, 30, 31, 32, 35, 42, 43, 49, 57, 64, 66, 67, 68, 69, 70, 71, 76
estrogen dominance, 30, 31, 42, 66, 67, 68, 69
exercise, 30, 62, 63, 64, 65, 66, 68, 75, 76
facial hair, 31
fasting, 53
fatigue, 12, 15, 27, 28, 29, 30, 64, 65
fats, 6, 7, 25, 38, 45, 56, 63, 72, 73, 74, 75
fiber, 49, 60, 62, 63, 68
fibroids, 57
FIR, 53
fish oils, 63, 68, 76
GABA, 30, 32, 65, 77
gallbladder, 30, 50, 69
GH, 31, 34, 42, 70, 71
glandular extracts, 64, 65, 66
Hashimoto's, 41
hCG, 54
heart, 26, 28, 30, 64, 65, 66, 67, 74, 70
heartburn, 60
homocysteine, 35, 68
IGF-1, 34, 42
immune, 27, 28, 58, 61, 63, 64, 65, 74
incontinence, 31
infection, 11, 34, 38, 57, 58, 61, 73
inflammation, 26, 31, 57, 58, 63, 64, 65, 68, 70, 72, 73, 74
insomnia, 27, 64, 75, 77
insulin, 26, 30, 35, 61, 62, 63, 65, 67, 68, 69, 70, 73, 74, 79

insulin resistance, 26, 61, 62, 69, 70, 73, 74, 79
iodine, 66
irritable bowel syndrome, 75
lead, 29, 30, 31, 32, 51, 54, 68, 75
libido, 31, 65, 66, 67, 70, 71
liver, 28, 52, 53, 54, 65, 69, 74
matrix, 9, 19, 36, 53, 54
memory, 28, 31, 32, 65, 75, 76
menopause, 28, 29, 30, 32, 68
menstrual dysfunction, 28
mercury, 11, 16, 17, 36, 37, 47, 48, 51, 55, 57
metabolic syndrome, 6, 7, 25, 26, 41, 61, 61
metabolism, 28, 30, 35, 43, 62, 68, 74, 75
mitochondria, 11, 15,16, 17, 18, 21, 22, 35, 44, 65, 73
mood, 32, 65, 68, 70
muscle mass, 31, 68, 69
neurotransmitter, 28, 30, 32, 66, 74, 75
omega-3, 11, 62, 63, 73
orgasm, 32, 70
osteoporosis, 28, 67, 70
ovary, 31
pain, 64, 75
parasites, 8, 22, 23, 24, 33, 38, 39, 50, 57, 59, 60, 75
perimenopause, 66, 67, 68
phosphatidylserine, 64, 65, 66
pituitary, 34, 41, 64, 65
PMS, 30
prebiotics, 61
pregnancy, 30
pregnenolone, 31, 66, 76
Premarin, 67, 68
PremPro, 68
probiotics, 59, 61
progesterone, 30, 31, 35, 41, 42, 66, 67, 68, 71, 76
progestins, 67, 76
prolactin, 35, 42, 67
prostate, 12, 14, 17, 18, 20, 25, 30, 31, 70, 71

protein, 52, 61, 63, 64, 69, 75
Provera, 67
receptor resistance, 34, 65, 66, 71
receptors, 29, 30, 31, 32, 63, 71
Reverse T3, 34, 41
selenium, 29, 51, 52, 60, 63
serotonin, 27, 28, 32, 65, 68, 75, 76
sex drive, 28, 32, 70
skin, 28, 51, 52, 53, 54, 68, 69
sleep, 26, 29, 32, 40, 47, 50, 61, 62, 64, 66, 70, 75, 76
soy, 66, 68, 75
stimulants, 27, 29, 32, 47, 75
stomach acid, 28, 60
stress, 26, 27, 28, 29, 30, 62, 64, 65, 66, 68, 71, 75
stroke, 30, 67, 68
T3, 29, 34, 41, 54
T4, 29, 34, 41, 54
testosterone, 29, 31, 32, 35, 42, 64, 69, 70, 71, 76
thermogenesis, 28
thyroid, 26, 27, 28, 29, 30, 32, 34, 41, 54, 66, 77
tobacco, 47, 75
toxicity, 9, 11, 16, 29, 30, 44, 47, 49, 50, 51, 53, 54, 62, 63, 66, 67, 68, 69, 73, 74
trans fats, 45, 63
transdermal, 68, 69
tryptophan, 75, 76
TSH, 34, 41, 66
tyrosine, 65, 76
vaccines, 58
Vitamin D, 52
weight, 12, 15, 26, 28, 29, 30, 32, 62, 75
weight gain, 12, 26, 28, 29, 30
weight loss, 28
Wilson's Temperature Syndrome, 41
wrinkles, 28, 31, 68
xenoestrogens, 14, 30, 31, 42
yeast, 8, 22, 24, 25, 38, 39, 40, 57, 59, 60, 61, 63, 78

www.ingramcontent.com/pod-product-compliance
Lightning Source LLC
Chambersburg PA
CBHW031300280526
45784CB00004B/1934